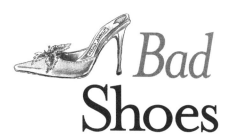

Bad
Shoes

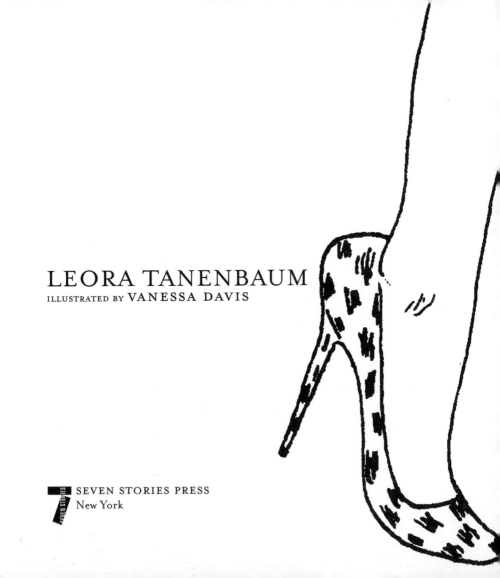

LEORA TANENBAUM
ILLUSTRATED BY VANESSA DAVIS

SEVEN STORIES PRESS
New York

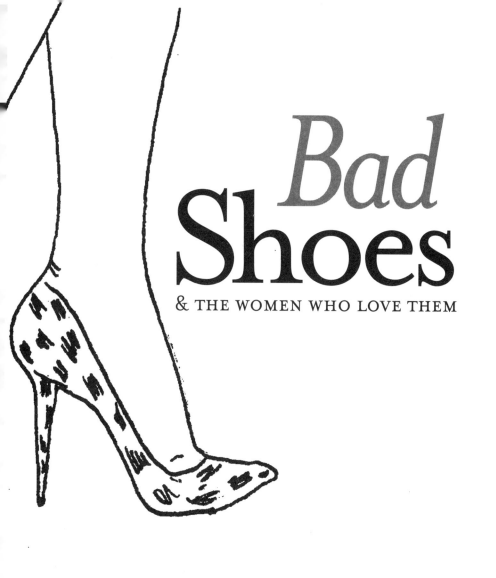

Bad
Shoes

& THE WOMEN WHO LOVE THEM

SEVEN STORIES PRESS
140 Watts Street
New York, NY 10013
www.sevenstories.com

In Canada
Publishers Group Canada, 559 College Street, Suite 402, Toronto, ON M6G 1A9

In the UK
Turnaround Publisher Services Ltd., Unit 3, Olympia Trading Estate,
Coburg Road, Wood Green, London N22 6TZ

In Australia
Palgrave Macmillan, 15-19 Claremont Street, South Yarra, VIC 3141

College professors may order examination copies of Seven Stories Press titles for a free
six-month trial period. To order, visit http://www.sevenstories.com/textbook
or send a fax on school letterhead to (212) 226-1411.

Illustrations by Vanessa Davis
Book design by Pollen, New York

Library of Congress Cataloging-in-Publication Data
Tanenbaum, Leora.
Bad shoes and the women who love them / Leora Tanenbaum, illustrated by Vanessa Davis.
p. cm.
ISBN 978-1-58322-904-0 (pbk.)
1. Shoes--Psychological aspects. 2. Women's clothing--Psychological aspects.
I. Davis, Vanessa. II. Title.
GT2130.T36 2010
391.4'13'082--dc22
2009052678

PRINTED IN THE UNITED STATES

9 8 7 6 5 4 3 2 1

Contents

Preface POP QUIZ
1

Introduction HEAD OVER HEELS
3

Chapter 1 BEAUTIFUL SHOES, UGLY FEET
9

Chapter 2 LOVE STORIES, HORROR STORIES
27

Chapter 3 WHAT YOU SHOULD KNOW FROM HEEL TO TOE
55

Chapter 4 TOETOX: Cosmetic Surgery of the Foot
75

Chapter 5 THE HISTORY OF HIGH HEELS
93

Chapter 6 THE SEX LIFE OF WOMEN'S SHOES
119

Chapter 7 SHOES WISELY: How to Shoe Shop
141

Notes
163

Index
173

NOTE TO THE READER
Please be aware that the author is not a medical specialist. If you are experiencing any
medical problem, you are advised to consult a trained medical professional—preferably
one who does not wear four-inch stiletto mules in the operating room.

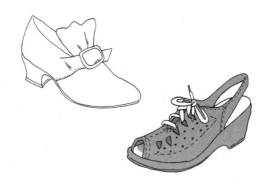

Pop Quiz
TRUE *or* FALSE?

1. Only radical feminists, granola-eating earth mammas, and wizened old ladies wear comfortable shoes.

2. Wearing high-heeled shoes on a regular basis can shorten the tendons in the back of your heels.

3. Wearing fashionable shoes can be a way to manage unconscious anxiety about gender and sexuality.

4. High heels were invented by men in an evil plot to subjugate women.

5. Ballet slippers are better for feet than heels.

6. Flip-flops are good when your feet hurt and you need a break from heels or tight shoes.

7. If you can wiggle your toes inside your shoes, you should go down a size.

8. If a woman wears high-heeled, pointy-toed shoes on a regular basis, in time the shape of her feet will become warped.

9. Sometimes shoes hurt a little in the store, but that is not a problem because you can break them in after you buy them.

10. Women have been warned about the dangers of wearing platform shoes and high heels for over 500 years.

Introduction

HEAD OVER HEELS

IT HAPPENED in Milan at a 2008 Prada fashion show. "I was having a panic attack, my hands were shaking," a runway model recalls. "Some of the girls were crying backstage, they were so scared." Why the dramatics—An act of terrorism? An explosion? Had the prime minister been assassinated? No. These women were fearful of walking down the runway in the season's extremely high heels. Two models tripped and fell; they were helped to their feet by members of the audience. One was so badly shaken she went backstage and never reemerged. The other finished her walk carrying her shoes and received a standing ovation.[1]

Since that day, models in strappy five-inch heels have stumbled at fashion shows presented by the designers Gucci, Miu Miu, Hervé Léger by Max Azria, Emilio Pucci, Dsquared2, and Rodarte. At a 2009 Brian Reyes show in New York, the pointy Manolo Blahnik pumps the models wore caused so many topples and were so uncomfortable that by the finale, *every* model was walking barefoot.[2] According to *Harper's Bazaar*, "the runways looked like an episode of *ER*."[3] In 1994, Naomi Campbell fell wearing nine-inch-heeled shoes during a fashion show of punk British designer Vivienne Westwood. But that had been a onetime event. Fifteen years later, models were dropping like flies. Meanwhile, models who rationally renounce menacing footwear pay a professional price. In 2009, several world-famous models refused to wear stilettos with ten-inch heels down an Alexander McQueen runway and were cut from the show.

If fashion models, who are paid to wear the creations of designers, cannot wear extreme heels, who can? Well, many ordinary women have been making a go at it over the last decade. Shoes with heels of five, six, even seven inches and bondage-themed straps are marketed to us as of-the-moment, edgy, and fashionable. These "bad" shoes are in the stores, and women are actually wearing them, not only in the evening when they go out to dinner, a party, or a show—but all day long. "Over the last several years," observes Jessica Morgan, who chronicles celebrity fashion faux pas on the Go Fug Yourself website, "we've seen designers creating increasingly crazy heels—shoes that runway models can barely walk in, and that we're scared to even wear out of the house for fear of taking a tumble at an inopportune time (like, say, in front of a bus). Regardless of the insanity of some of these shoes, we've still seen women whipped into a frenzy for them."

In June 2009, *Vogue* editor André Leon Talley, a regular front-row guest at designer fashion shows, demanded an end to the madness. After considering the ubiquitous "towering torture chambers, often poorly designed for the well-being of the foot," he declared, "I, for one, am over the mania for the high, high heel. Too many career women look like a herd of fashion beasts, aping one another in impractical shoes." Talley pointed out that women in previous generations knew how to look elegant without martyring their feet, and said that women today should reject designers' creations. "I do like to see women who know how to glide gracefully along on a sensible low heel."[4]

There is no denying the fact that when a woman is wearing "bad" shoes she gains sex appeal. Heels change your posture, making the body look more curvaceous because the pelvis and bust are forced to tilt forward to compensate for the shift in balance. Your legs seem longer, and your gait, sexier. There's a reason that sex symbols always wear heels.

Many women, at least some of the time, want to be sexually appraised. They want to feel sexy and they want others to judge them as sexy. Sometimes when they walk twenty city blocks to work, or push a stroller, or dash to the market for groceries, or enter a conference room, they imagine they are strutting down a runway. Life may be messy and hectic, but a little bit of appreciative physical attention can go a long way in boosting a battered self-image. High-heeled shoes are not comfortable. They are not practical. Often, they are not affordable. But a good pair of high heels can make a girl feel like a rock star.

And they had better. Any woman who has soaked her feet after a day's work, or bandaged up her bloodied heel, knows: stumbling is just one of the consequences of high-heeled shoes. They hurt. Sometimes, they hurt *bad*. What every woman *doesn't* know, however, is what I'm concerned about, and the reason I wrote this book. It's a fact: When worn on a regular basis, any shoe with a pointed toe and a heel over one and a half inches—let alone five—can cause foot deformity. In this type of shoe, the wearer is forced to walk on the balls of her feet, which leads to misalignment of the structure of the foot. In time, gorgeous shoes will create ugly feet, not to mention pain that shoots from the foot to the knee to the hip to the back.

In this book I explore the phenomenon of women choosing to wear "bad" shoes. Women love them despite the fact that medical evidence is unequivocal: they are physically damaging. And this is nothing new. Women in the West have been wearing "bad" shoes on and off for over five hundred years, while women in the East have been seduced by "bad" shoes for even longer. Trying to have a rational discussion with shoe-loving women, that they really ought to make more sensible footwear choices, is nearly always futile. But I'm here to make a plea. Feet are important. They will carry you around for the rest of your life. You need to take care of them.

To the reader who loves her high heels: My fervent hope is that when you finish reading this book, you will choose to reduce the amount of time you spend standing and walking in them. I'm not telling you to stop wearing them. I wear "bad" shoes too—but in moderation. Be smart about how often you wear them and for how long. If you wear them too much, you will end up with disfigured feet. And no one will give you a standing ovation for that.

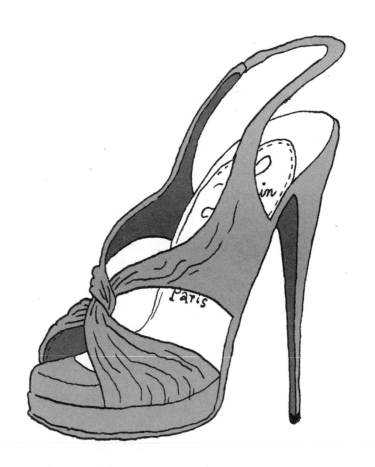

Chapter 1

BEAUTIFUL SHOES, UGLY FEET

IT WAS a Monday morning during the worst recession in US history since the Great Depression, but no one would know it the day I visited 1022 Shoe, the high-end, fantasyland designer shoe boutique at Saks Fifth Avenue in Manhattan. To get there, I hurried past the makeup counters on the first floor and dashed into the express elevator—the one that stops only on the eighth floor—just as the doors were sliding shut. A moment later I stepped out, and behold! I was greeted by a kaleidoscopic array of Christian Louboutin patent leather peep-toe pumps. One pair was robin's egg blue; the next was maraschino cherry red. Others beckoned in bubblegum pink, sunflower yellow, and seafoam green. Oh, and look over on the other side of the display—there was also an animal print option in shades of brown, beige, and black.

Jimmy Choo, Yves Saint Laurent, Chanel, Oscar de la Renta, Dior, Valentino, Dolce & Gabbana—the names don't really matter.

All the shoes in 1022 Shoe—the strappy sandals, the slingbacks, the closed-back pumps—looked more or less the same. The style formula of the season: high, thin stiletto heel; covered platform of an inch; pointy, open toe; colors that were bright, patent leather, metallic, and/or psychedelic. Sometimes a rosette or bow added an extra decorative touch. These shoes were gorgeous, extravagant, fantastical. They were works of art; they transformed the wearer into a princess, a sexy goddess.

And the prices—$695, $1,025, $1,575. Even if a woman could afford the price tags without blinking, the shoes were audaciously impractical. Who could stand in them for more than a few minutes, let alone walk in them? The heels were five inches high and so, so slender. The part of the heel that touches the ground was as wide in circumference as a single Cheerio. The words "hobble" and "cripple" popped into my mind. Even the boots were nonfunctional: most had open toes.

They were also oozing with sex appeal. The heels were so high and the shoes themselves so open and revealing, I imagined that only strippers and other sex workers could wear them without irony. These shoes looked like they belonged on the set of a pornographic video.

Yet dozens of women were not only milling around, they were trying on and purchasing multiple pairs. I sidled to two sisters in their twenties, tourists from

Australia, who were trying on Yves Saint Laurents. The pumps had five-inch heels. "How long can you wear them before your feet hurt?" I asked. "I can wear them all night," said one. Her sister nodded. Their mother confided, "I can wear them, but I can't walk around in them." Yet she was buying heels too. In fact, a good number of the shoppers were decidedly not young. Women in their sixties and seventies, with too-tight skin and hair impossibly blond, were pulling out their Saks cards as well.

My own feet encased in sporty lace-up shoes, I sat down. I leaned back into one of the mushroom-colored suede sofas and gazed at the chandeliers—clear glass bubbles suspended in cascades. I looked around, noticing that inside some of the display shoes there were foot mannequins. The dummy feet were realistically shaped, arches and all. Yet not one dummy foot fit into any of the shoes. The bottoms of the mannequin feet did not touch the inner soles and instead were awkwardly semi-suspended. But no matter. In real life, would-be Cinderellas crunch their toes and jam in their heels.

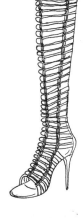

On my way out, I stopped and chatted with one of the salesmen. (Most of the salespeople were men, dressed in dark suits. Women buying fantasy stilettos apparently want men in dark suits to kneel at their feet, and are willing to pay obscene prices for the privilege.) He told me that the heels that season were the highest ever. But not to worry. He picked up a Louboutin and showed me that although the heel itself was five inches, there was a two-inch platform. "So in reality," he declared triumphantly, "it's only like a three-inch heel!" Even still, that's got to hurt and be hard to walk in without twisting an ankle.

Shoes have the power to transform an outfit from the mundane to the magical. High-heeled shoes give the illusion of elongating the legs, which is slimming. And shoes are relatively easy to shop for; you don't have to enter a dressing room and disrobe. For many women, myself included, that fact alone makes shoe shopping particularly alluring. So what if my toes squish just a little to fit, or if I get some cuts and bruises? Isn't that the price of being a woman?

I don't enjoy being the messenger of bad news, ladies, but you should be aware that your most fashionable high-heeled shoes, no matter how chic and status-laden, harm your feet. And it is not only high heels we need to consider. Flip-flops and ballet flats can be just as harmful as heels. Since the gladiator sandal trend rose up, sphinx-like,

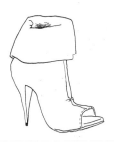

there have been lots of ankles encased in complicated straps and buckles. Don't be fooled. Pancake-flat shoes without arch support can make a woman feel like she's been fighting all day long in a Roman amphitheater.

But don't worry. There are still myriad captivating shoes out there that you can wear comfortably, safely, and femininely. By the time you finish reading this book, you will know all the tricks to look enchanting without suffering. You don't have to give up your fancy shoes, but you do need to be smart about wearing them.

It's okay to wear stilettos for a few hours once or twice a week at a party, date, or special event. I am not telling you to haul a bag filled with all your heels to the Salvation Army. Even if I did, you wouldn't listen. So keep your heels. But know this: it is foolish to wear them when you will be walking or standing for long periods of time, and it is downright dim-witted to wear them all day, every day, for years on end. If you choose to ignore these warnings, the day will come—maybe next year, perhaps in five or ten—when you will wake up in pain. You will look back at your years of bad decisions and wonder: "My god, what have I done?"

In *Sex and the City*, Carrie and her friends pound the Manhattan pavement in stilettos very similar to the offerings at Saks—shoes with itty-bitty toe boxes, zero arch support, inhumanly narrow foot beds, and a slope that forces feet forward so that you have no choice but to walk on the balls of your feet. For me, the mystery is not if they live happily ever after but whether or not they develop bunions (when the big toe shifts angle, pointing toward the little toes instead of straight forward) and hammertoes (when toes curl down), among other nasty afflictions.

Many of us recoil from the sight of orthopedic shoes because they are sexless, devoid of any style, and instantly add years to the wearer.

But guess what? By wearing shoes you associate with sex appeal and youth, you are actually uglifying your feet. It is paradoxical but true: in the pursuit of beauty, you are creating ugliness.

Every spring, when the temperature rises and children gleefully run out to parks and pools, millions of women look down and groan. They notice that their toes are misshapen; ugly corns have sprouted, and hey, what is that hideous bony protrusion on the base of the big toe? Instead of enjoying the freedom of sandals, many women cover up their feet with embarrassment. According to a 2008 American Podiatric Medical Association (APMA) study, more than 50 percent of women say their feet embarrass them "always, frequently or sometimes."[5]

"It is generally agreed that if you wore women's fashion high-heeled shoes with the narrow pointed toe box for up to ten years, you will end up with common foot deformities that are a direct result of the shoe," says Dr. Carol Frey, a leading researcher on the hazards of fashionable shoes on women's feet as well as an orthopedic surgeon in Manhattan Beach, California, and a clinical professor of orthopedic surgery at University of California—Los Angeles. "These conditions include bunions, bunionettes, pinched nerves, ingrown toenails, corns, and calluses."

Furthermore, many women fall so in love with a shoe style that they will buy and wear it even if it's too small. "Around eight years ago," one woman confides, "I had been eyeing a pair of Prada platform high heels with a zebra print and a hot pink bow on the front. They were insanely expensive and I couldn't justify spending that kind of money. Then they went on sale but only in a half size too small for me. So I bought them and squeezed my feet into them. They hurt but I wore them. I knew it was a bad idea, but I got so many compliments."

Often the shoe size technically is correct for a particular woman, but the style of shoe does not fit her feet properly because the shape of the shoe is unnatural. But that doesn't stop her. "I wore a pair of shoes the other day that were the right size but killed my feet," another shoe lover relates. "I wore them anyway, knowing that by the end of the day I would be in excruciating pain. The heels were around three inches and I walked around in them all day. They matched my dress perfectly. They are tweedy, grey and black, with a silk grosgrain ribbon. I will probably wear them again because they go so well with this dress."

Most women's fashionable shoes are shaped differently from women's unfettered, naked feet. Feet tend to be wider in front than at the heel, and toes do not naturally scrunch up to resemble the point of an arrow. Like most women, you probably have had no idea that wearing shoes with a shape that deviates from the shape of your feet is a recipe for disaster. After all, it's perfectly fine to squeeze your fanny into tight jeans: the worst that will happen is the sprouting of "muffin tops" above your waistband. You can change into a different pair of jeans, the muffin tops will disappear, and you can breathe again. Phew! But shoes are not jeans and feet are not love handles. Says New York

City podiatric surgeon Johanna Youner, "If you continue to wear a high heel, you will mold your feet into what a high heel looks like, but that is not what a foot is supposed to look like."

When it comes to fashion for feet, we must remember that bones, tendons, muscles, and ligaments are involved. The pressure of your body landing on your feet with each step is enormous. "Bottom line, the foot's primary responsibility is to be a shock absorber to the body's superstructure," emphasizes Dr. Rock Positano, director of the Nonsurgical Foot and Ankle Service at the Hospital for Special Surgery in New York City, and the foot and ankle consultant to the New York Mets and New York Giants.

Men and women alike need to take care of their feet to prevent problems, but women in particular need to wake up and smell the nail polish. According to a 2009 study by the APMA, far more women than

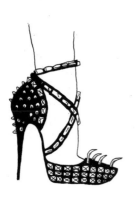

men—a whopping 87 percent versus 68 percent—suffer because of painful footwear.[6] Because of cultural expectations of femininity, only women feel pressured to endure pain on a regular basis. Only women are conditioned to believe that chronic pain is normal and the price of being considered attractive.

Women far outnumber men as foot surgery patients. A staggering 94 percent of all bunion surgeries are performed on women. Women also disproportionately go under the knife to correct hammertoes (81 percent), neuromas (89 percent), and bunionettes (90 percent).[7] Descriptions of these unsightly, uncomfortable, and sometimes unbearable conditions are found in Chapter 3.

My belief is that if a woman knows full well that wearing her favorite shoes may lead to hammertoes and bunions, and she makes this choice with informed consent, that is her decision. However, most women are not informed and therefore put their feet at risk for the sake of fashion and beauty without even realizing what they are doing.

In all seriousness, I suggest that pointy-toed, high-heeled shoes come with a warning printed on the shoe box, just as with cigarettes: "These shoes are a health hazard. Wearing them for prolonged periods on a regular basis may lead to deformity, pain, and ugly feet. Your Achilles tendons may shorten, making it impossible to wear flats even if you want to. Wear with caution."

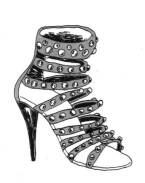

Many people mistakenly believe that the way celebrities live is attainable for the rest of us. But stars are not like us, even if paparazzi capture them at the market buying the same cereal we eat. Too many otherwise sensible women foolishly deduce that since Susan Sarandon gave birth at forty-six and Geena Davis at forty-eight, they too will be able to conceive beyond their peak reproductive years. Just because we see celebrities in stilettos on red carpets at award shows and premieres does not mean that the rest of us can or should wear the same shoes on a regular basis.

Today there is an urgent need to educate women to make smart footwear choices because of two current trends.

First, today many women consider extremely high heels to be an indispensable part of their wardrobe, and they don't just save these shoes for special occasions; they wear them all day, every day. High heels worn to work and around town are nothing new, of course, but now dizzying heights are taken for granted as "normal." In previous years, a three-and-a-half-inch heel was ooh la la. Now that height is categorized as "medium height" and women feel pressured to go as high as five inches.

When I visited the Jimmy Choo boutique on Madison Avenue in Manhattan, I picked up a pair of slingbacks with obscenely high heels (and no platform) and turned to the saleswoman. "Over five inches," she reported. "Can you walk in these?" I asked her. "*I* can't," she said.

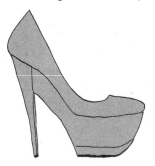

Another pair on display had a three-and-a-half-inch heel. "That's the medium-height heel," the saleswoman told me, without a trace of irony. "That one people can walk in."

Actually, even the three-and-a-half-inch heel is painful for many and treacherous for most. Yet this heel height is dismissed as child's play. The June 2009 "What's In, What's Out" page in *Harper's Bazaar* says it all: "In: Sky-high stilettos. Out: Mid-height pumps."

The new five-inch norm has been manufactured in large part by Christian Louboutin, the designer of signature red-soled shoes, currently favored by red-carpet celebrities. Few fashionistas know the pronunciation of his name, but that doesn't stop them from wearing his pornography-inspired stilts. (For the record, the correct way is KRIST-yen Lu-bu-TEN, with soft Frenchy "n"s). When I visited his Madison Avenue boutique, some of the heels were—I am not making this up—over six inches high. I couldn't decide which was more obscene: the height or the price. Marked down on sale, most of the styles were being sold for $657 (from $1,095).

What I find most surprising about the trend to go higher and higher is that it flies in the face of common sense after September 11, 2001. Among other horrible images from that day, I vividly remember the women in downtown Manhattan who had worn heels to the

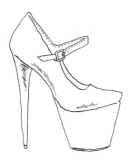

office. In desperation, they took off their shoes and fled barefoot. This extreme case exposes the impractical reality of many women's shoes. Aren't shoes supposed to offer mobility, or at least not inhibit it?

I asked the question of Elizabeth Semmelhack, chief curator of the Bata Shoe Museum in Toronto and author of *Heights of Fashion: A History of the Elevated Shoe*. She also finds the trend counterintuitive. In 2001, Semmelhack had just completed a timeline charting the history of the high heel through the centuries. "The last shoe I put in was from Tom Ford. It was very fetishy with a very high heel. Then September 11 happened. Women were quoted saying that they would never wear heels again. I wondered what the next shoe would be on the timeline. I was fully expecting a flat. But there was no hiccup at all! There was not a moment in which women embraced a common-sense approach to footwear. It never happened."

Another trend is the widespread enthusiasm for flip-flops. Over the last decade, flip-flops have become a staple in the wardrobes of women, men, children, and adolescents. Even high-end designers such as Chanel and Manolo Blahnik manufacture them. It is estimated

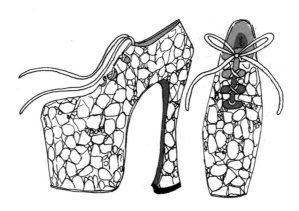

that 220 million pairs costing more than fifteen dollars (in other words, excluding the rubber pairs sold in drugstores) are sold each year.[8]

Many women turn to flip-flops because their feet hurt after hours in heels. They mistakenly believe that flip-flops are like medicine to soothe their aching feet. They could not be more wrong. The lack of support in this type of sandal causes the foot to move and roll, leading to multiple injuries and problems, such as the painful heel condition called plantar fasciitis. Since flip-flops remain fashionable and trendy—with millions choosing to wear them when walking and even bicycling—it is critical that women be educated about the damage they are doing to their feet. Flip-flops belong at the beach or pool, and for a half-hour after a woman paints her toenails and isn't going anywhere anyway—and that's it.

YOU MIGHT be thinking, "What does this Leora Tanenbaum person know? I bet she wears sensible Eleanor Roosevelt shoes. I bet she is an earth-mamma feminist who has never felt the rush of wearing breathtaking stiletto platform peep-toes." So let me fill you in. I love beautiful heels too, which is what led me to write this book. I'm not a "back to nature" type by any imaginative stretch. I eat healthfully but

I also enjoy red meat. My husband, who loves hiking, pulls my arm to join him. Yes, I'm a feminist. But guess what: feminists are not opposed to beauty or pleasure. I enjoy getting made up and dressed up. I've been known to wear Spanx beneath my wrap dresses.

Allow me to share my own story. A year ago, my feet and knees started to hurt even when I wore flats or sneakers. It got bad enough that I visited a podiatrist, who informed me I had bunions. *Bunions?* The word made me think of onions and bad breath. It turned out that my pronated feet (they roll inward), which I always thought had no consequence other than my walking a little ungracefully, are a health hazard.

According to the podiatrist, my shoes did not cause my bunions—I can thank heredity for that—but they exacerbated the problem. From that moment on, he pronounced, I was to wear customized orthotic inserts with arch support in all my shoes, sandals, and boots. He did not recommend surgery, although many bunion sufferers do go under the knife. In a haze over the expense of custom orthotics—which insurance companies do not reimburse—I was delayed in my realization that I was in for a big lifestyle change. Trendy shoes, especially mules and slingbacks, do not accommodate orthotics. I've never been a fashion plate, but I certainly never expected that before hitting midlife I would be cruising the grandma aisle at the shoe store.

Bunions are no fun. This is my cautionary tale. But don't take my word for it. Listen to the medical experts.

"The human body was not designed to walk on three-inch or four-inch heels, which produce severe anatomical distortions and can result in orthopedic problems from the lower back down to the feet," writes Glenn Copeland, the consulting podiatrist to the Toronto Blue Jays and the author with Stan Solomon of *The Good Foot Book: A Guide for Men, Women, Children, Athletes, Seniors—Everyone*. "High-heeled shoes put abnormal stress on the back of the leg, the knees, and the lower back."[9]

Warns the American Orthopaedic Foot & Ankle Society (AOFAS), "[P]revalent forefoot deformities including bunions, hammer toes, claw toes, corns, neuromas and bunionettes are associated with the repetitive use of ill-fitting shoes."[10]

"I tell my patients to save their pretty shoes with four-inch heels for dinner in the evening and not to wear them for more than two hours," Dr. Youner tells me. "They shouldn't walk more than the distance from the car to the restaurant. I have a patient who fell off her four-inch heels in January and was in a cast until May. She broke a lot of bones across the midfoot and across the center foot. It was very bad and she had to do physical therapy. It can be very dangerous to wear these shoes."

"I never tell people, 'Don't wear a high heel,'" agrees Dr. Positano. "I'm not an opponent to heels. I'm just an opponent to wearing them in situations that are not optimal. I say, 'Don't wear a high heel if you're going to be walking two miles or standing for five hours.' People get into problems when they don't wear their shoes judiciously. When you're wearing a high heel, you put more stress on the muscles, the tendons, the ligaments, the bones."

I asked Dr. Positano if it's inevitable that a woman who wears heels on a regular basis will develop foot problems. "It's a Russian roulette thing. You can keep pushing the trigger, and maybe nothing will happen for a long time," he told me. "But eventually something will happen."

According to a 2003 survey conducted by the APMA, women are walking around in a lot of pain because of their shoes.[11] The findings will make you want to throw a stiletto at the window of your favorite shoe store:

- Nearly three-quarters (72 percent) of women wear high heels, with 39 percent wearing them daily.
- Nearly three-quarters (73 percent) of the women reported experiencing physical problems caused or aggravated by wearing shoes.
- High-heel shoes are worn one to four hours a day by 20 percent, and five or more hours a day by 19 percent, of women. Ten percent wear heels more than eight hours a day. Ouch.
- The most common foot conditions are blisters (36 percent), pain in the ball of the foot (35 percent), and corns and calluses (29 percent), followed by pain in the arches of the foot (26 percent), heel pain (23 percent), ingrown toenails (16 percent), and bunions (15 percent).

- Most women (62 percent) wear heels two inches or higher.
- A large majority (72 percent) reported that they have had to stop wearing some kind of shoe because of a foot problem.

If you step back—assuming you're able to with the shoes you're in—you can't help but wonder if American women shut down their brains while shopping for shoes. AOFAS has published a statement that "foot problems resulting from poorly fitting shoes have reached epidemic proportions and pose a major health risk for women in America."[12]

I've had some time now to scope out the selection of footwear called "comfort shoes." In truth, the choices aren't quite that limited. Many companies now create shoes with support that aren't ugly, some that are even a little cute. Each season the stylishness increases a notch, so I'm hopeful for the future. Many shoes also have insoles that can be removed, creating space for orthotics. I do wear high heels without orthotics once or twice a week, but only for a few hours at a time and I never do serious walking in them.

We all know that looking feminine can be painful—from plucking, waxing, chemical peeling, and injecting. Whether or not we accept or reject this situation, we can all agree that a woman should not damage her body permanently in the pursuit of looking attractive. For those of you reading this book who have healthy feet, I beg you to protect them now while you can. Pluck and wax if you must. But choose your shoes wisely; don't let ill-fitting shoes cut off the circulation of blood to your brain.

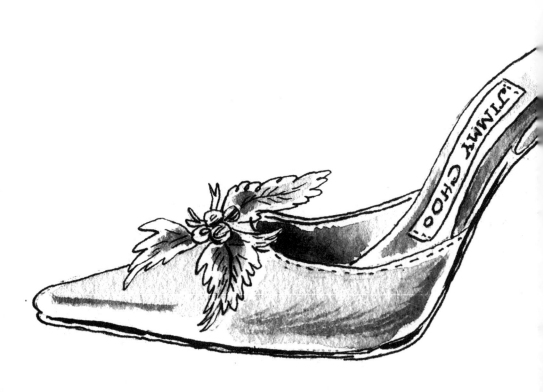

Chapter 2

LOVE STORIES, HORROR STORIES

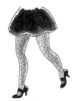

"I'M A shoe person," women who love shoes are wont to say. "I'm into shoes." Or: "Shoes are my thing." If they're under forty-five, they confide, "I'm a real-life Carrie Bradshaw." If they're over forty-five, they tell me, "You should see my closet. I'm just like Imelda Marcos."[13]

It is telling that ordinary women feel an affinity with larger-than-life figures known for their gluttonous collection of gorgeous shoes. Shoes hold a mystique for women that other articles of clothing do not. Unlike dresses or skirts or blouses, shoes hold their shape even when no one is wearing them, and therefore evoke a sense of promise. When you see a pair of stilettos on display in a department store or featured in a fashion magazine, you can imagine yourself wearing them and becoming the kind of person who lives a magical life, gliding around gracefully with no need for sensible, lace-up shoes.[14] The fantasy just might become realizable by stepping into the shoes and inhabiting them.

Very often, what women "love" about shoes is this *frisson* of poten-
tiality, of expectancy. When considering a beautiful or unusual pair of
shoes, whether high heeled or not, they think: *This is what I could be. If I wear
these shoes I will become a new me—a better me—a me whom others will recognize as fear-
less and exciting. No longer will I be a woman who plods and clunks along. In these shoes I
can be fun, edgy, sexy, unpredictable. Anything is possible.*

Alas, as we know, the fantasy is never truly attainable. Gorgeous
shoes do not lead to a carefree life, or even to the appearance of one.
A classic example is Dorothy in the film *The Wizard of Oz.* In the L. Frank
Baum novel on which the film is based, her shoes are silver, but in the
1939 movie they are memorably red-sequined. As long as Dorothy
wears her dazzling ruby slippers she lives in a fairy-tale world in which
she wants no part because she misses home. When she returns to the
reality of her Kansas life, her feet become shod in practical oxfords.

The most didactic (and gory) morality tale about conspicuous shoes
is surely "The Red Shoes" by Hans Christian Andersen. In this 1845
story, an impoverished orphaned girl named Karen is so taken with a
pair of red shoes she is charitably given that she can think of nothing
else, even when in church taking communion. Karen refuses to con-
form to religious and social norms, which dictate humility and mod-
esty. The villagers condemn her for her vanity. Red shoes are sexually
provocative and symbolize her desire to assert her own will. As pun-
ishment, her shoes become fixed on her feet and force her to dance
without stopping. Karen becomes physically exhausted and can't con-

tinue in her state. In despair, she begs an executioner to chop off her feet, rendering her an asexual, dependent cripple who hobbles on crutches. She begs forgiveness from her Creator, and her soul flies up to God.

Clearly, sexually provocative shoes can symbolize female willfulness, freedom, and power. These stories echo a belief held by many women that wearing gorgeous shoes can be a magical and empowering experience. Carrie Bradshaw, the *Sex and the City* character played by Sarah Jessica Parker who spent all her money on designer shoes, is invoked repeatedly when I ask women who love shoes why exactly they love them. It is worth analyzing what she represents: a woman who tries to wrest control of her identity, her sexuality, and her image through her shoes. Her dream is to become successful in love and life, and she believes that her shoes will make her dream come true.

One episode of the HBO program is always mentioned. In this episode, titled "A Woman's Right to Shoes" (obscenely suggesting that shoes are as important to women as reproductive choice), Carrie goes to the baby shower of a friend, Kyra, played by Tatum O'Neal. As always, Carrie has spent considerable time and effort to coordinate a sexy and fashionable ensemble. On this occasion she is wearing high-heeled Manolo Blahnik d'Orsay sandals (a style in which the sides of the shoe are cut away, leading to a very revealing look) with rhinestone buckles. Upon arrival at the shower, held in Kyra's apartment, Carrie (along with all the other guests) is instructed to leave her shoes in the foyer so as not to track dirt inside the home. She's not happy about the situation—her shoes are the centerpiece of her outfit and the item sure to get attention—but she is obedient and slips them off.

A few hours later, after the shower is over and Carrie is preparing to leave, she returns to the foyer—only to discover that her beloved, bejeweled shoes are missing! Someone has stolen her Manolos! Kyra does not show any empathy. She loans Carrie black, androgynous, worn-in canvas sneakers to wear home. In the following days, Carrie continues to be disturbed about her loss and pesters Kyra to see if the shoes turn up. They don't. Carrie has hundreds of other pairs of shoes, but she feels incomplete without this particular pair. Kyra offers to replace them for her, but is aghast and judgmental when she discovers that Carrie's shoes cost $485. To Kyra, that is an irresponsible amount of money to spend on shoes for oneself. Kyra determines, therefore, that she is not responsible for replacing such an extravagance.

Carrie wonders if Kyra is correct. Perhaps she has made an existential error in choosing the single, childless lifestyle (in which she doesn't have to spend money on anyone but herself) instead of Kyra's traditional path of husband and babies. Ultimately, Carrie rejects this interpretation. Since she has always been a loyal friend who buys gifts for others when they marry and give birth, she decides that she, too, is deserving of gifts. Carrie registers for her missing shoes at the Manolo Blahnik boutique, in effect announcing that she is marrying herself, and leaves a message on Kyra's machine to let her know. Kyra then purchases the shoes off the registry. When Carrie receives them, she is ecstatic. She has her shoes back; she has her life back; she has her sexual identity back. Her life choices are as valid as Kyra's, even though they are not the conventional ones.

Within the context of the show, we are expected to identify with Carrie and regard her as an empowered woman who writes her own life script. Kyra is so condescending that it feels good to root for Carrie, who refuses to be bullied. If she chooses to throw away her money on frippery, well, that is her right! "I related to Carrie," a woman who wears expensive heels herself said to me. "Why was it so irresponsible for her to buy designer shoes? The Tatum O'Neal character"—who is clearly affluent—"was probably spending $900 on her European stroller, so why couldn't Carrie spend $500 on shoes?" I would add that if Carrie's shoes were sturdy and orthopedic but just as expensive, they would not have been regarded as excessive, but rather as a necessity. It is their sexualized impracticality, combined with their price tag, that make the shoes offensive to Kyra.

But seen from another angle, Carrie is a desperate, disempowered character and her shoe collection underscores this point. True, Carrie has positive characteristics—she is exceedingly loyal to her friends; she is kooky and creative and thoughtful—but ultimately, as watchers of the TV show and the movies know, she is highly self-involved and seeks personal satisfaction and empowerment through commodities. It's no accident that her closet is filled from floorboard to ceiling with luxurious, high-end, fantasy shoes. Carrie's heels represent to us that she is unable to plant her feet firmly on the ground. Her eyes flit around in the clouds; she is unable to see the truth: that the love of her life may be willing, finally, to marry her, but that he is not a dependable person. It is doubtful that he is capable of being loyal to her.

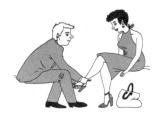

Why do women love shoes?

I SPOKE with fifteen women, ages twenty-five through seventy-four, and asked: Why do you love shoes? Here is what they reported:

Shoes are easy to shop for:
"You don't have to go into a changing room."

"You can find a great pair in fifteen minutes."

"When you've been pregnant and your weight has gone up and down, you don't always know what size clothes you should buy and which size will fit you a year from now. But with shoes, you know your size."

You can wear them the same day:
"Clothes need to be altered. With shoes, you can put them on right away and enjoy them immediately."

High-heeled shoes are sexually alluring:
"You walk differently in heels than you do in sneakers. If they're open and reveal your toes, you feel almost naked."

"Wearing high heels is a very simple way to feel womanly. I recently became comfortable wearing sexy shoes to the office and just out and about. I used to have the mentality that you only wear heels when you go out at night. But I work at a fashion blog and I can get away with dressing in a womanly way, so I do."

"I met my new boyfriend three weeks ago because of a pair of shoes. I had just gotten paid for the month. I went to J. Crew and fell in love with a pair of five-inch heels. They are brown with an ankle strap and a strap that goes across your

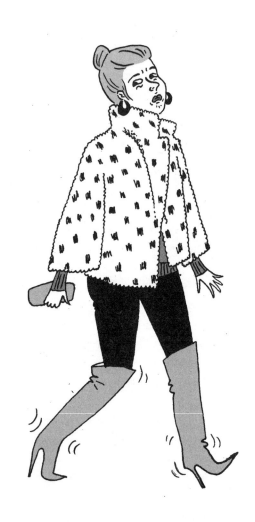

toes, but you can't see that strap because it's covered by a big piece of golden fabric scrunched up in a flower shape. They are really pretty and can match with anything. I am usually a very cautious shopper but I fell in love with these shoes. They cost $250, which is the most money I've ever spent on any single item. They were a big deal for me. I wore them right away to a party. Right after I got there, one guy said to me, 'I love your shoes.' Then several other people, some guys and a girl, said, 'What great shoes!' Then one of the guys asked me to put up my leg so that he could see the shoe better. It was embarrassing but a funny way to start a conversation with people I didn't know. One of the other guys held me to keep my balance. And now he's my boyfriend."

"My husband and I have been together for twenty-two years. We've gone through periods where we're too busy and too tired to have sex. One day he was so desperate and I made a joke that he should pay for it. I said, 'Okay, for a nice pair of shoes or boots.' That was my bargaining chip. He handed me the money and the next day I went out and picked the pair myself. I'm not joking. I exchanged sex for a new pair of shoes. And I've done it several times. I make him pay up front. He puts the money on the dresser. It's now up to a thousand dollars. Did I just say that out loud?

[laughter] I am willing to get a red bottom so that I can buy shoes with a red bottom. [laughter] The truth is that I've spent the money not only on shoes but on stuff for the kids. [laughter] I've gone to Bloomingdale's and bought $500 shoes that were on sale for $300. I've also bought a pair of boots. The thing is that when I wear them, all day I think about the sex. It changes my gait because I'm thinking about being with him. I know the story behind it, and only I know the story behind it."

If a woman is dissatisfied with her body, at least she knows that shoes can always make her look good:
"Shoes don't make my ass look fat."

"When you get older, you become shorter. So I want heels to compensate for my loss in height."

Shoes can make a woman stand out from the crowd:
"You shouldn't look like everyone else. People say, 'Well, if I'm going to spend a lot of money on shoes, I'll buy a basic black pair that I can wear with everything.' But I think the opposite. If I'm going to splurge on one pair of shoes, I would buy purple. They would make a statement. Last year I bought a dress that was orange with hot pink

pockets. I was with my friend, who said, 'Now you have to go and get shoes.' And I said, 'Don't worry, I already have hot pink shoes!'"

"I worked in a corporate office for eleven years. No one there seemed to care about clothes or have any fashion sense. But I feel that when you put yourself together and look polished, you are received well by others—especially when you are a woman in a corporate workplace. So I always wore nice outfits to work. It got me noticed. Luckily I had substance to back myself up. But wearing nice clothes and especially nice shoes were a way to separate myself from the pack of people."

"I love to wear shoes that are colorful. It shows that I have spunk. It shows that I have character."

"If I buy an interesting dress, I can't wear it twice in the same week. But if I buy a pair of edgy shoes, I can wear them every day. People expect you to wear the same shoes over and over, so you get more for your money."

Expensive shoes are a sign of status:
"They're like driving a BMW."

Shoes are life markers:

"I keep all the shoes that have memories for me. I have the shoes I wore for my sweet sixteen, the shoes I wore at my wedding, the shoes I wore on my trip to Russia, the shoes I wore when I met my husband's family the first time. I organize my memories around the shoes I was wearing."

"When I was in my twenties, I would window-shop on Madison Avenue. One afternoon, as I did my usual gaze into the Charles Jourdan window, I spotted a quilted shoe with a patent cap toe and a chunky mid-level rubber heel. It screamed dressy, casual, suit, dress, walkable, danceable, young, and über-chic. I figured one splurge wouldn't change my finances, and the shoe was from the company's cheaper line, Bis, anyway. I slipped them on and was in love. I purchased them in black with a black cap toe and wore them for the forty blocks home. I was at the store the next day, even before the shop opened. I bought them in every color scheme—cream with black toe, navy with navy toe, red with red toe. I knew I had 'arrived' when the clerk said that the store would deliver for free to my apartment. I wore them every day. I wore them hiking, to a black-tie wedding, with beach attire, to work. Every photo from the time I was twenty-three to twenty-seven I was in those shoes.

I felt so hip and well dressed wearing them. However, when I would take them off there would be a terrible toxic smell. It was so awful that it permeated the room. How could something so beautiful smell so bad? I took the shoes to a shoemaker who diagnosed the stench as coming from cheap glue trapped in the insole that led my sweat to combust into an olfactory weapon. Soon after I went to Paris and continued to wear my favorite shoes when I was sightseeing. But at the end of the day, when I returned to my tiny hotel room, I was blown backward by the smell. My other pairs of quilted cap-toe shoes that were in the room were creating this horrid condition. Sadly, I packed them all up in a plastic laundry bag, tied an airtight knot, and threw them in a trash bin on Avenue des Ternes."

REAL WOMEN report that the actual experience of owning fantastic shoes inevitably falls short of the fantasy. It's not often that women find their shoes stolen from a friend's apartment, as Carrie does, but it is very common that they become disappointed with their purchase and might even be better off if they *were* stolen. This is because shoes such as Manolo Blahnik d'Orsays are unbearably uncomfortable for more than a short period of time. It's hard, if not impossible, to keep the fantasy going when you've got blisters and need to duck into the nearest drugstore to get more Band-Aids because the ones you've been wearing are losing their adhesiveness and are threatening to spill over the side of your shoe as a badge of shame. Few women admit when their shoes are uncomfortable because that would mean admitting the fantasy is not achievable. If they admit the truth, they have wasted their money and let their dream slip away. They are made to be a fool. And yet, inexplicably, they go out and buy impractical beautiful shoes . . . again and again.

Even Sarah Jessica Parker herself has conceded that in her real life, she has trouble wearing stilettos. "I used to spend eighteen to twenty hours a day filming in heels," she told the British edition of *Elle* magazine in 2007. "Now I spend a much shorter day in them and I'm like, 'Owww!' I've really destroyed my body by running and dancing in heels. My knees are shot.'"[15]

It's no wonder, then, that Parker has been seen walking around downtown Manhattan in comfortable shoes. (Those cobblestone streets are brutal on your soles.) She was excoriated in the fashion blogosphere in March 2009 when she was spotted several times in a pair of bizarre-looking designer boots that were cloven-toed. Instead of one toe box there were two, dividing the big toe from the other toes.[16] Could it be that Parker was trying to protect a bunion? And if the actress portraying the Cinderella-esque Carrie can't tolerate heels, who can? Is the fantasy achievable for *anyone*?

The answer: no, it is not. When you wear beautiful but uncomfortable shoes, your feet *hurt*. Cinderella's feet didn't hurt because her shoes—albeit glass—fit her properly. And who knows? Maybe those glass slippers had a contoured foot bed.

A New York City mother of two young daughters, Janet, told me how excited she was when she received a gift of Jimmy Choo heels—her first pair of luxury shoes. She had befriended a woman at her children's preschool, Julie, and the two of them joked about Manolos and Jimmy Choos. Janet didn't realize it, but her new friend was not just joking around. She was very affluent and actually owned many pairs of shoes from these designers. The day before Janet's birthday, Julie had her personal shopper from a trendy boutique called Scoop deliver a pair of Jimmy Choos to Janet's apartment.

"So I open the box," Janet tells me. "Inside were these incredible shoes. This woman had bought me gold Jimmy Choo heels! I didn't think I could accept such an extravagant gift. I tried to give them back to her but she just said, 'Enjoy them; just think of me when you're enjoying them.'"

"But here's the thing," Janet continues, getting serious. "The pair she had bought me weren't my size. They were a 7 and I'm a 7.5. So I went to the store and explained that I needed a size larger. But they didn't have any left in any size. But then I saw that the store had another pair that I loved even more—but only in a size 6. So I exchanged my pair for that pair. I have to shove my feet in them. I love them. They are the sexiest things. They are very strappy. I can't walk around in them but I did wear them to a show, when I took a taxi there, and I wore them once to a wedding. My feet kill when I wear them. But the fact is that even if they were my size, they still would never be comfortable. The heels are very high and one of the straps cuts right over the bunion area, and the other straps dig into my skin."

A suburban woman, Carol, tells me about a professional conference she attended in Atlanta. She knew that many elegant women would be in attendance, and she wanted to look her best. On her flight, there was a tornado. "Everyone was feeling jangled," Carol recalls. "The plane was circling the airport. The woman sitting next to me had white knuckles. Then, all of a sudden, in the middle of this tornado, I realized that I had forgotten to pack my dress shoes for the dinner I had to attend that night. I only had the sneakers I was wearing on the plane. I couldn't decide which was worse—the tornado or not having shoes?

"So when we finally landed, I found a shoe store in the airport. It was a Bally store and the shoes were much more expensive than any shoes I'd bought in my life. But I felt that I had to buy something because I couldn't wear sneakers to the dinner. So I bought a beautiful but simple pair of black pumps. The salesman said, 'Don't worry. The more you wear them, the less they cost you per wearing.' I said to him, 'No kidding! Then I'm going to sleep in them!' But in the end, I only wore them that one time, that evening. They hurt too much. When I got back home I had them stretched but they still squeezed my feet."

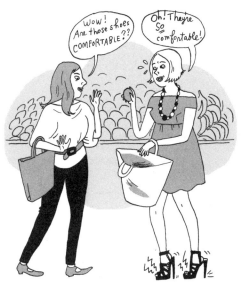

"But Are They Comfortable?"

WHEN A woman asks another woman if her shoes are comfortable, this is not friendly, idle chitchat. Far from it. This is a coded, loaded message: "I recognize that you are putting vanity before comfort and practicality. I am onto you. You can't fool me!" If the first woman answers, "They're comfortable, really!" is she lying? Is she suggesting that she's not as vain as she appears? I asked several women if they ever lie. Their answers reveal that while they sincerely *want* to answer truthfully, they also want to maintain the fiction of comfort to justify wearing their bone-crunching shoes. Here is how they explain themselves:

"I used to wear four-inch heels every day to work. I did it for over fifteen years, and last year I had a baby so now I wear mostly flats. People would ask, "Are they comfortable?" and I would always say, 'They're not uncomfortable.' And that was the truth."

"Every time I put on my fabulous black high heels I feel great because I like the way I look in them and I like the attention I get. I get a huge reaction but it's not usually from men. It's always from other women. I don't lie. I say they are not that uncomfortable. I say they are worth it. I am consciously making a cost-benefit decision. My shoes aren't comfortable, but neither are they painful. I can't walk that far in them, but I freely admit it. The discomfort is a price I'm willing to pay for feeling fabulous."

"I hate it when women claim that they are comfortable even when it's clear that they are not."

"The problem is that usually I don't know the shoes will be uncomfortable because they feel okay in the store. By the time I realize they hurt, it's too late. So what am I supposed to do? It's not like I want to wear shoes that hurt. But that's too much to explain."

"If someone asks me if my heels are comfortable, I tell the truth. 'No, but they're pretty.' Or, 'Can't you see the Band-Aids on my heels?'"

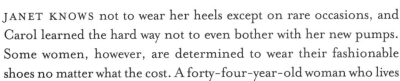

JANET KNOWS not to wear her heels except on rare occasions, and Carol learned the hard way not to even bother with her new pumps. Some women, however, are determined to wear their fashionable shoes no matter what the cost. A forty-four-year-old woman who lives on Manhattan's Upper West Side, Olivia, works in the fashion industry. The names inside her shoes are Chanel, Manolo, Prada. "I don't wear heels every day," she says, because they slow her down. Also, one of Olivia's heels tends to hurt because of a bone spur (a not-uncommon phenomenon in which there is extra bone growth on the heel, caused by aging and/or poorly fitting shoes, discussed in the next chapter). "I have to calculate my lead time when I'm wearing heels. It takes me longer to get to work when I'm wearing them. They drag you down and you can't just be on the go. When there was a transit strike a few years ago, I walked to work in sneakers and changed when I got there, but that's not my thing, so after the strike was over I stopped with the sneakers."

Olivia shares with me a revelatory story to demonstrate that she had reached the point of no return—at least on one particular day. An observant Jew, she walked over to her synagogue, just a few blocks from her apartment, on a recent Sabbath morning. She wore "these cute Prada heels, maybe two and a half inches." Her plan had been to just go home after synagogue. But it was a beautiful day so instead of going straight home, she decided to take a walk in Central Park.

"But after a little while my feet hurt, and it got to the point where I just couldn't pretend anymore. I took off my shoes and walked barefoot in the park." Olivia does not carry money with her on the Sabbath and therefore could not resort to an emergency taxi ride home. "But then I had to leave the park to get on the street. There's a difference between being barefoot in the park and being barefoot in the street. So I decided to put my shoes back on. But then I realized, who was I kidding? They hurt too much and I couldn't do it. Besides, my feet were filthy now and even if they didn't hurt I didn't want to put them back inside the shoes. But I really couldn't imagine walking around in the streets barefoot. So I wiped the bottom of my feet with my sweater and put my feet back in my shoes. It was really painful."

"So next time," I ask, "will you bring comfortable shoes with you in case something like this happens again?"

"No!" Olivia replies with an unspoken suggestion that I have not been listening carefully. "The shoes were not all that high! They were open-toe and they just put too much pressure on the balls of my feet. It's not like I wear four-to-five-inch-heel shoes. I only buy shoes that are comfortable in the store, always less than three inches. I'll keep wearing heels as long as I can. I don't want to walk around in comfortable shoes. The only time I'll do it is when it's raining. Then it's a great excuse."

I don't want to walk around in comfortable shoes. Olivia says this as if wearing comfortable shoes—i.e., well-made shoes that fit her properly—would be the height of humiliation. In her mind, wearing comfortable shoes is equated with "ugly" shoes (which is absolutely not true, but we will get to that later), and wearing ugly shoes is not an option. She believes that despite the pain, she must wear a certain type of shoe. She believes that she does not really have a choice.

The question is: *Does* she have a choice? Or is Olivia at some level pressured—coerced, even—to wear excruciatingly uncomfortable shoes?

Today's feminist rhetoric of "choice" when it comes to women's adornment is a response to the radical feminism of the 1960s and 1970s. Before the women's liberation movement, American women were expected to wear skirts, girdles, garter belts with stockings, makeup, and—let's not forget—high heels when they were at work or in the public eye. We owe a huge debt of gratitude to "women's libbers" for insisting that these beauty standards are part of a larger system of discrimination in which women are regarded as lesser than men.

In 1968, they protested the Miss America pageant. In the leaflet the New York Radical Women handed out in Atlantic City, they argued that "women in our society are forced daily to compete for male approval, enslaved by ludicrous 'beauty' standards we ourselves are conditioned to take seriously." At the pageant there was a huge "freedom garbage can" (linking their agenda with the civil rights movement's "freedom rides") into which protestors threw symbols of beautification—eyelash curlers, girdles, curling irons, and home permanent kits.[17]

Millions of consciousnesses were raised: Wait a minute, liberated women said to themselves and to each other, this girdle is oppressive! So are these false eyelashes! And so is this lipstick, and these high heels. Into the trash they go!

Many other women, of course, were never persuaded that they were being oppressed at all, while others were ambivalent: They liked looking feminine in their miniskirt and mascara, but maybe not every day. They didn't want to be told that they must dress up, but when they did it on their own terms they enjoyed it.

In the 1980s, consumer choice was touted as a form of citizen empowerment. A new form of liberal feminism developed, championing women's role as market consumers to "choose" whether or not to participate in beauty practices. By the 1990s, the editors of a magazine called *Bust* were telling young feminist readers that women have the power to choose whether or not to be sexually objectified. Coeditor Marcelle Karp weighed in:

"[A] woman's choice to mold her body does not make her a victim. If bigger boobs are what she wants, it's her right to choose both as a feminist and as an individual. . . . We BUST girls are not immune to feeling insecure about our bodies, but we're smart enough to know that we don't need to be victimized by it."[18]

Concurred Debbie Stoller, *Bust's* other coeditor:

"Unlike our feminist foremothers, who claimed that makeup was the opiate of the misses, we're positively prochoice when it comes to matters of feminine display. We're well aware, thank you very much, of the beauty myth that's working to keep women obscene and not heard, but we just don't think that transvestites should have all the fun. . . . We love our lipstick, have a passion for polish, and, basically, adore this armor that we call 'fashion.' To us, it's feminine, and, in the particular way we flaunt it, it's *definitely* feminist."[19]

This new feminist credo of the 1990s was that women have the power to exercise personal power and therefore to "choose" to bare their bra straps and to get an eye lift if that is what they want to do. This "girl culture" was supposed to be a form of feminine strength and power. It's okay to flaunt your femininity, young women were told, as long as they were culturally hip, ironic, and knowing enough to recognize that they were referencing RuPaul and not Donna Reed.

The truth lies somewhere between the beauty trash can and the Botox parties. Most of us do have significantly more leeway to "choose" whether or not to wear eye makeup than women did before the Miss America protest, but let's not get carried away: women in America continue to face enormous pressure to appear feminine. If we deviate from this cultural norm—with or without irony—we pay the price. A bare face, an outfit that hides the body, and those dreaded "sensible" shoes are markers of a woman who refuses to play the game. In some communities and neighborhoods, women routinely say no to flirty, feminine frocks without an eyebrow raised. But in others, a woman who resists the social pressure to dress in a stereotypically feminine way opens herself up to ridicule. Many Latina women, for example, report that they feel pressured to wear high heels (*tacones*) as a way to celebrate their heritage.[20] Women of all ethnicities who are anxious about being considered too "masculine"—regardless of their affectional orientation—may also feel a pressure to wear heels and dresses so as to disguise an appearance they worry is not sufficiently feminine.

So are women *really* making a free "choice" when they wear shoes so uncomfortable they have to take them off and walk barefoot? When standing in front of her closet and deciding whether to wear her loafers or her heeled pumps, a woman flips through a mental cache of images of the different ways her body will appear physically and also the different ways she will appear on the femininity scale. Does she want to be judged on that scale, or does she want to step off of it? Most would rather be judged and given approval than ignored or mocked. Therefore women like Olivia wear shoes that seemed comfortable in the store but are excruciating on the street. It's true that no one is twisting anyone's arms—although if they wear platforms, they may twist their own ankles—but most women who are compelled to wear impractical shoes feel pressured to prove or display their femininity.

Paradoxically, many women believe that high heels can signify strength. Everyone knows they hurt, so the wearer is clearly not a weakling, and they cause the calf muscles to become defined, emphasizing the wearer's musculature. For the comedian Sandra Bernhard, wearing high heels is about proving her toughness. "When I walk out the door in a good pair of heels," she told the *New Yorker,* "I never feel vulnerable, there's no time for any weakness, I feel focused strong secure, my stride is potent and no one hassles me when I'm on the corner hailing a cab. . . . Because I demand respect and my heels back me up."[21]

I surmise that Sandra Bernhard has a potent stride in any footwear she slips on. She believes that her heels have a transformative ability to confer respect, but I doubt this is the case. They make *her* feel "focused strong secure," which no doubt affects her posture, her manner, and her strength of mind. In the end, wearing shoes we love is an exercise in transforming *ourselves*, not those around us.

Let's not fool ourselves: fabulous shoes don't give us power. In fact, the opposite can occur. Stephanie, a twenty-five-year-old woman from Connecticut, remembers a few years ago when she went out with some friends to a jazz club. She was dating a musician at the time, John, and he had joined them. Stephanie borrowed a pair of "crazy high platform boots" from one of her friends. "The heels were six inches, maybe higher. The boots were fake leather and zipped to above the knee and they had these giant platforms. They were really something else. I had to hold onto my friend when I walked. It was just a fun thing to do. I remember that when John saw me in the boots, he smiled at me. I can remember exactly how his face looked when he smiled."

Later that night, after Stephanie and her friends had returned to one of their apartments, one of the guys said to her, "Those are some crazy shoes. John thought they were *ridiculous*." At that moment, Stephanie realized that John had been making fun of her behind her back. She had assumed that when he had smiled at her, it had been a smile of appreciation or approval—that she looked outrageous in a quirky, attractive way. But no. He thought she looked like a fool. "After this guy told me that, I felt ashamed. John must have thought I would do anything to get people to look at me."

"I remember buying the most expensive, beautiful, caramel-colored Italian leather boots with pointed toes and three-inch heels when I was twenty-two," remembers Mary Marcdante, a Del Mar, California–based women's health speaker and founder of BunionSurvivor.com. It was thirty years ago and Marcdante was on a trip to New York City. "If *Sex and the City* had been on the air then, Carrie Bradshaw would have stopped me on the street and wanted to know who I was. I felt beautiful, powerful, smart, and sexy—for about fifteen minutes of imaginary fame. I wore them walking (and crying) for three hours. Even today, I wince in pain remembering the raw and bleeding blisters I created wearing them. But I loved them. I loved them so much that even though I chose to no longer wear them—because, as they say about relationships, when the pain outweighs the joy you eventually let go—I turned them into a fashion sculpture and kept them as a bedroom doorstop."

We like to imagine that if we wear fashionable shoes, others will perceive us as strong, sexy, and in control. But when a woman is a slave to fashion, it is quite likely that others regard her as a victim of her own making. Is that really worth the price of a case of Band-Aids and corn pads?

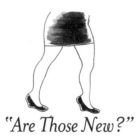

"Are Those New?"

Confides one shoe lover, "I used to buy a new pair of shoes and then go outside to scuff the bottoms so that my husband wouldn't know I had new shoes. If he asked if they were new, I would just show him the bottoms and say, 'These are so old!'"

Women across the land are clued in to this trick. Reports another, "I used to hide my shoes from my husband when they were new. Then when I would wear them I would be like, 'Oh, you're just noticing them now.' He thinks it's a sickness [to keep buying new shoes], and he isn't wrong."

Chapter 3

WHAT YOU SHOULD KNOW
FROM HEEL TO TOE

DO YOU ever really look at your feet? Can you visualize what they look like from all angles, not just from the top? If not, put down this book, remove one of your shoes, and take a look. Notice that the bottom of your foot is not flat: it curves to form an arch toward the inner side, with open space beneath the arch. Now look inside your shoe. Chances are, unless you happen to be wearing running shoes or "comfort shoes" today, the insole does not rise to fill the open space beneath your foot's arch. Your shoe, therefore, does not match up to the shape of your foot. (Even if your shoe has a heel, if you removed the insole it would lie flat.) This means that your shoe does not have what is called "arch support." A shoe with arch support has an insole that lifts to fill the open space beneath the arch of the foot, offering a customized fit.

Strange, isn't it? Your jeans follow the contours of your waist and behind and legs; your shirts are fitted to your shoulders and bust and waist. If your clothes did not follow the lines of your body you would

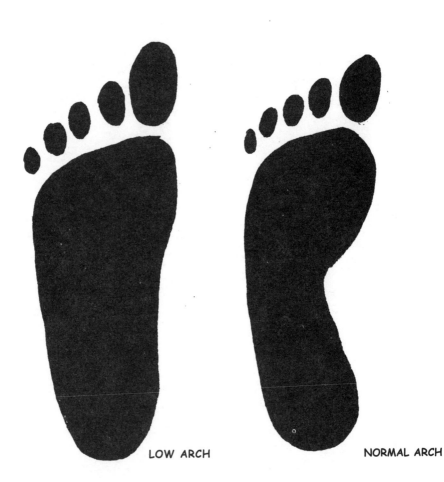

LOW ARCH

NORMAL ARCH

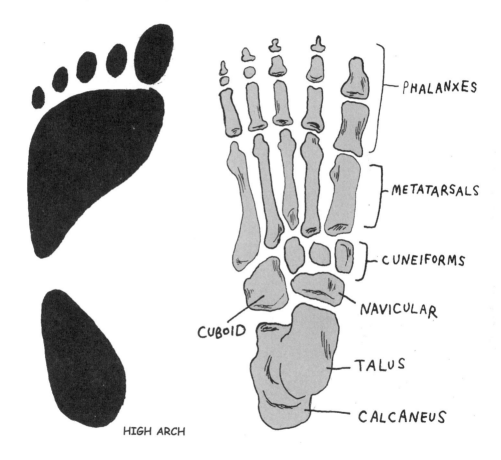

HIGH ARCH

PHALANXES

METATARSALS

CUNEIFORMS

NAVICULAR

CUBOID

TALUS

CALCANEUS

take them to a tailor or save them for a sloppy day of housecleaning. Shouldn't your shoe complement the shape of your foot?

If we all walked barefoot, we would not need arch support because our feet would function normally. Feet don't actually *need* shoes. But since we grow up wearing shoes to protect our feet from sharp, hard, and unsanitary objects, our feet become compromised: our muscles weaken, our toe alignment shifts, our joints become restricted. It is ironic that shoes, which we wear to protect our feet, cause our feet to function improperly. "Imagine if someone put a cast on your arm when you were three years old and you never took it off," explains journalist Adam Sternbergh. "Your arm would stop working. That's kind of what's happened with our feet. . . . Shoes perpetuate shoes. It's a classic self-perpetuating system."[22]

Some lucky people manage just fine: their feet are in good shape and they can get by with a lack of arch support. But most of us—up to 70 percent of us—walk with excessive pronation, meaning that our feet roll inward more than they should. Those of us who pronate too much develop problems eventually. When a pronator wears a shoe lacking support, her foot moves around too much and an abnormal amount of force is placed on her forefoot. Over time, this pressure leads to foot disorders.

Women tend to pronate more than men, according to Dr. Carol Frey, a leading researcher on the causal relationship for women between wearing poorly fitting shoes and developing foot problems. We also have smaller Achilles tendons. Since our feet and ankles are different in structure and biomechanics (the way they move) from the feet and ankles of men, we in particular must be careful to wear shoes that have arch support and fit properly.[23]

With each step we take, the body lands with pressure equal to one-and-a-half times its weight. Over the course of a typical day we take between five thousand and ten thousand steps, so the impact on our feet is tremendous. The average person absorbs over a million pounds of step impact through her feet every day.

To enable us to withstand this level of pressure, our feet are brilliantly constructed. One quarter of all the bones in the human body are contained in the feet, with each foot boasting twenty-eight bones. The skin on the bottoms of our feet is twice as thick as the skin on the rest of our body, and it is joined with a special plantar fat pad that provides cushioning. ("Plantar" means "having to do with the sole of your foot.") There are over a hundred joints, tendons, muscles, and ligaments holding the foot together.

With each step, certain parts of the foot are flexible and other parts remain rigid. All the structures work together to enable the foot to create an arch that collapses and springs back. The plantar fascia, the longest and strongest ligament in the body, runs along the sole and stretches and contracts like a rubber band. Meanwhile, our body weight is transferred from heels to toes. When everything is moving as it should, we can walk, run, and jump without a second thought. Now take another look at your foot. Twist it around. Rotate it at the ankle. Bend your toes. Remarkable, isn't it? This is definitely something you want to take care of.

With normal gait, the foot strikes the ground at the heel, then rolls forward and inward toward the arch and toes. If the foot is flat, too flexible, and rolls too much, it "overpronates." If the foot is too rigid, with a high arch, and doesn't roll enough, it "oversupinates." The overwhelming majority of biomechanical foot problems—98 percent—are caused by overpronation, according to Dr. Glenn Copeland.[24] If your feet, knees, or back hurt, the culprit is often your gait. Your feet are not properly aligning and balancing your weight when you walk because of overpronation or oversupination.

If this is your situation, your doctor may prescribe either custom-made orthotics or over-the-counter shoe inserts. Orthotics and inserts allow the wearer to distribute pressure properly and improve balance. They alter the angle at which the foot strikes the ground during walking or running. They relieve discomfort and the symptoms of many foot conditions, and can prevent a number of problems from occurring in the first place. A person with a biomechanical imbalance should wear an orthotic or insert as much as possible.

If you are experiencing foot pain, the first thing you need to know is that *this is not normal.* Never assume that foot pain is something you just need to learn to live with. You don't.

If you don't have any foot discomfort at all, you're at a huge advantage. But don't congratulate yourself just yet: you must take steps to ensure that you don't develop any problems. Here are the most common problems affecting women who wear fashionable shoes on a regular basis.

BUNIONS

THIS IS a misalignment of the joint of the big toe. Health care specialists often refer to this condition as "hallux valgus," which is a fancy way of saying that the joint of the big toe (hallux) is bent outward (valgus). It is the most common foot disorder among women. The base of the big toe enlarges and angles toward the second toe instead of facing straight ahead. It's caused by abnormal pres-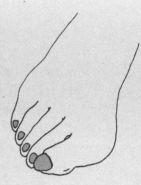sure placed on the big-toe joint because of excessive pronation and ill-fitting shoes. There is also a genetic component: a history of bunions tends to run in families.

If you do nothing to stop the bunion, it will progressively worsen, with the big toe angling further and further toward its neighboring toe. It's nice that your toes are such good friends but bunions are ugly and can become inflamed. They may be accompanied with hallux limitus (arthritis of the big-toe joint) or hallux rigidus (when the big-toe joint becomes rigid). They also hurt when they rub against the side of your shoe. Although it's not as common as the big-toe bunion, it's possible to develop a "bunionette," a bunion on the baby toe, also called a "tailor's bunion."

To avoid bunions: Unfortunately, for some people it may be impossible to completely avoid bunions. But you can slow down their development, and perhaps even stave them off, by wearing shoes with arch support (or orthotics or over-the-counter inserts) and with a roomy toe box. If your feet pronate, save your heels for once in a while rather than wearing and walking in them every day.

To treat bunions: Wear shoes with a wider space at the toes. Some shoes can be stretched at the site of the bunion so that the material of the shoe doesn't rub against it. See a medical professional to determine the best course of action. Wear an orthotic or over-the-counter insert. Wear a toe spacer between the big toe and second toe, a bunion shield, or a bunion splint to relieve the pressure. If all nonsurgical options have been exhausted, you might consider surgery, but be wary of promises from surgeons who promise a quick recovery. Get a second and third opinion. Potential complications include joint stiffness, infection, scarring, and swelling. If you surgically remove a bunion but continue to wear shoes that don't support your feet, the bunion can recur.

HAMMERTOES

A HAMMERTOE is a deformity in which the joint of one of the middle toes is bent and the toe therefore resembles a small hammer inside a piano. This occurs as a result of years of wearing shoes in which the toe is forced to squeeze into a too-small toe box. Over time, the toe fails to spring back to its natural straight position when it's released from shoe prison and becomes stuck in this unnatural, enslaved position. In a severe hammertoe, it's not only bent but also crosses over the toe next to it. If one of the two smallest toes develops into a hammertoe, it not only bends but rotates under slightly. It's possible to have more than one hammertoe on a foot.

By itself, the hammertoe is ugly but painless. However, it can cause pain because its existence changes the way the forefoot distributes pressure, which leads to corns, calluses, blisters, and inflammation of the joint. It also may rub against the shoe, which can lead to bursitis (inflammation of a bursal sac).

To avoid hammertoes: Don't wear shoes that put pressure on your toes. This means not wearing most high-heeled shoes and any shoe with a cramped toe box.

To treat hammertoes: Wear shoes with extra depth in the toe box. See a medical professional to determine the best course of action. You can buy over-the-counter pads, splints,

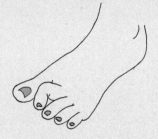

and toe sleeves to protect the painful areas. In severe cases, surgery may be necessary, but it's best to exhaust all nonsurgical options first, since surgery of the foot can result in complications that may be worse than the hammertoe itself.

CORNS AND CALLUSES

IF YOU'RE eating while you're reading, I advise you to put down your fork now, since you may lose your appetite. A corn is a hard, thick patch of skin found on the top of your toes or between them. No doubt you guessed that its memorable name derives from the fact that it looks like a kernel of corn. A corn develops because of undue friction: the toes rub together or against the shoe and the skin creates the corn to act as a buffer to protect itself. This often occurs because there is a hammertoe. By itself the corn can result from wearing shoes that are too narrow or too tight. A callus is a thick patch of skin that builds up on the ball of your foot, generally in response to too much weight pressing down on the metatarsal bones (the bones in the forefoot that sit at the base of the toes), often from wearing high-heeled shoes.

To avoid corns and calluses: Wear shoes that fit properly. The toe box should be deep enough and wide enough to allow your toes room to wiggle. If you must wear high-heeled shoes, don't wear them exclusively: alternate with low-heeled shoes. Buy heeled shoes with extra padding in the metatarsal area, or add foam cushioning in the forefoot of your shoes.

To treat corns and calluses: Same as above: change your shoes. See a medical professional to determine the best course of action. She might trim the corn or callus (you should never do this yourself). Over-the-counter corn pads are available but avoid medicated pads, which have acid that can burn the skin. If corns and calluses don't go away, you probably need orthotics or over-the-counter inserts.

PLANTAR FASCIITIS

PRONOUNCED: *Plant-R Fa-she-I-tus.* This condition causes sharp heel pain that usually presents itself first thing in the morning when you get out of bed and stand for the first time after having had your feet elevated. If that happens to you, it means that your plantar fascia is overstretched, injured, or inflamed. Plantar fasciitis is often confused with heel spurs, an overgrowth of bone in the heel, but heel spurs are actually a response to plantar fasciitis.

Plantar fasciitis affects women and men in equal numbers, and is seen in both the athletic and the sedentary. Factors that may lead to its development are being overweight or gaining weight; excessive pronation; wearing shoes without arch support; exercising more than usual or engaging in any physical activity in which you impose excess pressure on your heels; standing for long periods on a hard surface; or just getting older and having the plantar fascia lose much of its elasticity.

To avoid plantar fasciitis: Wear shoes with arch support, especially when walking or exercising.

To treat plantar fasciitis: See a medical professional to determine the best course of action. An injection of cortisone is available for immediate relief, but cortisone shots have side effects. The same is true with oral anti-inflammatory drugs. Other treatment options are physical therapy and icing the area. None of these treatments will eliminate the underlying problem, though. The best plan is to switch to shoes with proper support. This does not mean wearing shoes with extra cushioning, because extra cushioning can worsen the condition by allowing the arch to collapse.

MORTON'S NEUROMA

NAMED AFTER a podiatrist, this nerve condition is quite treatable despite its ominous-sounding name. Morton's neuroma occurs when there is an enlarged nerve between the third and fourth toes that causes a burning sensation or numbness in the toes. It is also referred to as a "pinched nerve." It is most common among women with wide feet who wear high heels and/or narrow shoes.

To avoid Morton's neuroma: Don't wear shoes that are too narrow for your feet. Don't wear shoes with high heels, since they require you to transfer your weight to the front of your feet, putting too much pressure there.

To treat Morton's neuroma: Wear shoes that fit properly. Wear an orthotic or over-the-counter insert to balance your feet properly

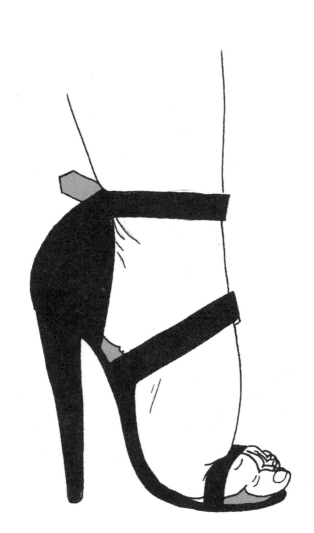

while walking. If the pain is severe, ask your doctor about padding, anti-inflammatory drugs, or cortisone injections for immediate relief, but be aware of side effects.

KNEE, HIP, AND BACK PAIN

WHEN YOU wear shoes with heels of one-and-a-half inches or more, you are forced to walk in an unnatural position. You place uneven pressure on the ball of your foot and the normal function of your ankle is compromised. The knee and hip are forced to adjust themselves to maintain stability. In short, your entire system of alignment and balance is out of whack, which can lead to chronic pain in your knees, hips, and back.[25]

I suffered from chronic knee pain and never suspected that it had anything to do with my feet. Neither did my general practitioner, who theorized that it was caused by a breakdown of cartilage. She may be right in part, but once I began wearing orthotics, my pain subsided nearly completely.

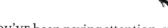

IF YOU'VE been paying attention, you now know that *if you don't wear shoes that fit properly, you are asking for trouble.* This is as clear as a Lucite heel if you read the medical literature. Wearing shoes with a narrow toe box and high heels can lead to bunions, hammertoes, corns, calluses, plantar fasciitis, and neuromas. They can also lead to less severe but also painful blisters and ingrown toenails.

To avoid or alleviate foot pain, switch to better shoes that do not force your foot into an unnatural position or shape. Otherwise, over time your naked foot will come to mimic the unnatural position or shape of the shoe, which is not only highly uncomfortable but also horrifying to look at.

A landmark study for the American Orthopaedic Foot & Ankle Society in 1993, coauthored by Dr. Carol Frey, demonstrated that almost all women wear the wrong shoes.[26] There were 356 healthy participants between the ages of twenty and sixty. Among her findings:

- Eighty-eight percent of the women in her study wore shoes that were too small.
- The average woman wore shoes that were too narrow by a half inch and too short by a half size or full size.
- Eighty percent reported significant foot pain while wearing shoes.
- Seventy-six percent had foot deformities, with bunions and hammertoes the most common.
- Fifty-nine percent wore uncomfortable shoes every day.
- Seventy-nine percent had not had their feet measured in the last five years when buying shoes.

Even the women in the study who did not have pain or deformity wore shoes that were too small. "The average woman in our survey, when asked what her shoe size is, reported herself as a size 8B," Frey told the *New York Times.* "But when we measured her foot at the widest point, right at the ball of the foot, we found that she is actually an 8C."[27]

In a follow-up study two years later, Frey and her colleagues revisited 255 of the women who had participated in the original study. Incredibly, a whopping 86 percent of these women—who at this point should have known better—continued to wear shoes that were smaller than their feet. This is only two percentage points fewer than in the original study. Frey and her colleagues know that these women's shoes were too small because they traced the subjects' feet (while standing) and compared the measurements with those of the subjects' shoes. Unsurprisingly, nearly three-quarters (73 percent) stated that they had some foot pain. Sixty-nine percent had one or more foot deformities: 71 percent of this group had bunions; 50 percent had hammertoes; 18 percent had bunionettes; and 17 percent had other deformities.[28]

It's hard to read this material and not want to track down these women and shake some shoe sense into them. *Hello?* You participated in an orthopedic study in which it was revealed that your foot pain is caused by wearing too-small shoes; it's two years later and you're *still* wearing too-small shoes?

By the way, it's not just women under the age of sixty who are so foolish. Another study of women and men over the age of sixty-two found the same result: they also wear shoes that are too small.[29] Older is not necessarily wiser in the world of footwear.

The thing is, the phenomenon of wearing shoes that are too small is not entirely due to poor shoe choices. Frey's research reveals that most women, especially pronators, have feet that are wide in front but narrow at the heel. However, most shoes are not constructed with a wide-enough front and narrow-enough heel. Women with this foot shape are stuck: do they choose shoes that fit in the heel or in the toe? If they wear shoes that are wide in front, chances are the heel will also be wide, and the shoe will slip off when they walk. As a result, most women are forced to compromise. Rationally, they choose shoes that grip their heel, even though this means that the front is too snug. Better to wear a too-tight shoe that stays on the foot than a wide shoe that falls off, they figure.

Most of us need shoes that are significantly wider in front compared with the back. These are called "combination-last" shoes or wide-sized shoes. However, the majority of fashionable shoes are only somewhat wider in front: the toe boxes are too narrow. The "last" of most shoes (the wooden or plastic form around which a shoe is shaped) does not match most feet. Even still, women are not off the hook. If we demanded more wide-sized shoes and shut our pocketbooks in protest of the ubiquity of narrow shoes, we could get more shoes made from realistic lasts into the stores.

Manufacturers create shoes more slim than wide because they know that women want their feet to look dainty. But this is lazy design. It is indeed possible to create flattering shoes that fit properly. Let us not reward manufacturers that insult us with designs that are beautiful but impractical and harmful.

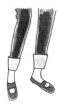

Exercise Your Feet

THERE ARE exercises you can do to strengthen your toes, lessening pain today and staving off more pain in the future. Dr. Frey has a detailed toe-strengthening program she recommends to her patients:

Big Toe Pulls

If you have bunions or toe cramps, wrap one thick rubber band around both big toes and pull the big toes away from each other toward the smaller toes. Hold for five seconds and repeat ten times.

Toe Pulls

If you have bunions, hammertoes, or toe cramps, put a thick rubber band around all the toes on one foot and spread the toes. Hold this position for five seconds and repeat ten times.

Golf Ball Roll

If you have plantar fasciitis, arch strain, or foot cramps, roll a golf ball under the ball of your foot for two minutes.

Marble Pickup

If you have pain in the ball of your foot, hammertoes, or toe cramps, place twenty marbles on the floor. Pick up one marble at a time with your toes and put it in a small bowl. Continue this exercise until you've picked up all twenty marbles.[30]

Dr. Frey also recommends toe stretchers such as YogaToes. She encourages everyone to take off their shoes and walk in the sand at the beach whenever they get the chance, because this massages the feet and strengthens the toes.

Meet the Specialists

Podiatrist

A specialist in the medical care of the foot, ankle, and lower leg. A podiatrist attends podiatric medical college and earns a doctor of podiatric medicine (DPM) degree. The American Podiatric Medical Association (APMA) is the leading professional organization of DPMs.

Orthopedist

An MD who attended medical school and is a specialist in problems relating to bones, joints, and muscles throughout the body. The American Orthopaedic Foot & Ankle Society (AOFAS) is the premier organization of orthopedic surgeons who are foot and ankle specialists.

Pedorthist

A nonmedical specialist who recommends foot devices and footwear to relieve foot problems. A certified pedorthist (CPed) has gone through special training and certification. Some shoe stores employ a pedorthist whom you can consult when choosing shoes for purchase.

Chapter 4

TOETOX
Cosmetic Surgery of the Foot

SOME WOMEN are so smitten with their shoes that even when experiencing excruciating pain, they refuse to give them up. In extreme cases, rather than change the shoe to fit the foot, they change the foot to fit the shoe. In today's age of extreme makeovers, why *not* snip off a piece of bone to shorten that pesky, long toe? In this world of liposuction and radio-frequency procedures that supposedly tighten sagging skin and reduce cellulite, why *not* get the feet to look as good as the rest of one's sculpted body?

Indeed, in the early 2000s, women started going under the knife either to fit into their narrow, pointy shoes or to make their naked feet look more streamlined. The procedures include removing a piece of bone in a toe to shorten it, fixing a bunion that doesn't hurt to remove the bump, and the injection of filler into the ball of the foot to add a layer of cushioning.

Although she is by far not the only doctor who performs these types of cosmetic foot surgery, podiatrist Dr. Suzanne M. Levine has been most willing to speak with the media about it. "Take your average woman and give her heels instead of flats, and she'll suddenly get whistles on the street," Levine told the *New York Times*. "I do everything I can to get them back into their shoes."[31] She added that she is "simply fulfilling a need, a need to wear stylish shoes." She herself models the trends, appearing on the *Today Show* in heels with witchy-looking pointed toes. The number one problem her patients cite is that other doctors tell them to stop wearing high heels, and they don't want to hear that. So instead they come to her to receive the message they do want to hear.

Vogue has called Levine "the podiatrist to Manhattan's A-list" and a "diehard Manolo wearer herself."[32] Her clients include Anna Wintour, Katie Couric, Diane Sawyer, Oprah Winfrey, and Barbara Walters.[33] "I'm not a proponent of doing surgery just to fit into shoes, that's not where I'm coming from," she told the *New York Observer*. "But I want to give women the opportunity to wear heels because they're going to do it anyway." She lamented that too many women listen to their other doctors and actually do make the switch to undangerous shoes. These women have had "several face-lifts, a nose job, their neck done, their lips enlarged a little too much and lo and behold you look down to discover your grandmother's feet! It's shocking. On top, they're wearing a Chanel jacket and orthopedic-type shoes on the bottom. It's not very *sexy*."[34]

Levine runs a "medical spa," blurring the lines between medicine and cosmetic pampering. She calls it the Institute Beauté, and she runs it together with Dr. Everett Lautin, who specializes in Botox injections. According to the spa's website, Levine's "objective is for every patient to feel their best and return to their favorite pair of shoes as soon as possible," which is achieved through surgical procedures such as "toe shortening" and "foot narrowing."[35]

But after undergoing these surgeries, many patients go right back to their old doctors to try to undo complications from surgery that may not be undoable. The American Orthopaedic Foot & Ankle Society (AOFAS) warns patients not to undergo cosmetic surgery on the foot unless they experience pain or limited function because they risk complications such as infection, nerve injury, prolonged swelling of a toe, and even chronic pain with walking.[36] Over half of the society's members report that they have treated patients with problems resulting from cosmetic foot surgery.[37]

Dr. Rock Positano increasingly is asked to correct mistakes made by other surgeons. "It's scary," he tells me. "When a foot operation does-n't go well, it affects the person's quality of life in a way that they never expected. It baffles me when patients come to me and say, 'I had this surgery done. I wanted to shorten my toes and I wanted to remove that bump and I wanted to fit into nicer shoes.' And the end result is usu-ally, 'Now I have a problem that I didn't have before.' I see this all too often. Once you remove bone or change the alignment of the foot or the architecture of the foot, it is never quite the same. And we're not just talking about the foot. The foot has a direct relationship with how the lower leg, the knee, the hip, and the back work."

"But what if the patient is in pain and does need surgery, but as an added bonus can end up with a nicer-looking foot?" I ask. "Why is that a problem?"

"That's when people get into trouble," he says. "A patient goes into surgery that is medically indicated. For example, they have severe arthritis of the big toe and it's very painful. But then they say, 'Well, while I'm at it, why don't I remove a neuroma or a piece of bone off the hammertoe?' I see this so many times. It's the 'throw it in while you're at it' scenario that gets people into more trouble than you can imagine."

I know it's important to distinguish between purely cosmetic and medically indicated procedures. "But," I press, "what if there's an overlap? Is it so terrible to make your foot look nicer if you need surgery anyway?"

"Let me make this clear," Positano says. "When you need a foot operation, when you are in severe pain and you have exhausted all conservative methods, then you are a good candidate for surgery. But nine out of ten of the patients who come to this office do not need the surgery. The one patient who does need it inevitably does very well. That is because there is a psychological component. That patient was in severe pain and had exhausted all nonsurgical options. That patient went into the procedure with a better outlook on what would happen."

Dr. Sharon Dreeben, an orthopedic surgeon in La Jolla, California, and a former chair of the public education committee of AOFAS who has spoken out against cosmetic foot surgery, similarly emphasizes that the patient's outlook is critical. "When you *need* surgery, for the most part the benefits outweigh the complications," she explains. "When you don't need surgery because you're not having any pain, because you're able to walk and you have no true deformity, then the complications become greater than the benefits. I have had patients with real deformities, and that is a different issue. But when you have a thirty- or forty-year-old woman who wants to have her toes shortened so she can get into her Manolo shoes, she has an abnormal psychological profile of herself. Clearly the problem here is not the foot, but the brain."

Positano and Dreeben spoke to me in absolutes, but I was not convinced. There seemed to be a gray zone. Bunions and hammertoes are ugly but usually painless in very wide shoes. However, in shoes that are not orthopedic, they rub against the inside of the shoe and do become painful. So is correcting bunions and hammertoes in order to wear nonorthopedic shoes always a bad idea?

"There is no gray zone," Dr. Johanna Youner, a Manhattan podiatric surgeon, tells me emphatically. "You do not change the cosmetic appearance of your foot because you don't like the way it looks. You change it because it hurts. If you need the surgery and there is a cosmetic benefit, that works for everybody and everybody is happy. But you have to be careful. Some doctors will do the surgery when there isn't a lot of pain, and that can cause permanent discomfort. This is not a joke. There is no guarantee that everything will be perfect. If you shift things around you can end up with horrible trouble."

According to these doctors, and in the words of Positano, "nine out of ten" patients do not truly need the surgery. But when I speak with Levine, she tells me the opposite. "Nine times out of ten it *is* medically indicated," she says. (Doctors love to begin a sentence with "nine times out of ten.") She says she does not understand why the surgeries are controversial. "Toe shortening" is "nothing more than an orthopedic procedure. It's called arthroplasty. You shorten the toe for a hammertoe. It doesn't make sense" that this is condemned. "Foot narrowing," meanwhile, is "nothing more than getting rid of a bunion and at the same time you are narrowing the foot. In layman's terms, it's just getting rid of the bunion."

"By using the language of 'toe shortening' and 'foot narrowing,'" I ask, "aren't you confusing people?"

"Podiatrists are now performing traditional surgery but they are minimizing scars. What's wrong with that?" she asks. "But it behooves them to make sure that the purpose is to alleviate pain. You can't bill the insurance company if it's not medically indicated."

I ask Mary Marcdante, owner of the excellent website BunionSurvivor.com, about choosing bunion surgery to alleviate pain but with the added benefit of leaving the doctor's office with nicer-looking feet. "I've spoken with hundreds of women about their bunion surgery concerns, and one of the top comments is always wanting their feet to look better so they can wear prettier shoes," she tells me. Marcdante herself had long been ashamed of her large feet with "green bean toes and golf-ball old-lady bunions." Finally, she couldn't take the pain any longer and had the bunion removed on her right foot. "While I didn't ask for prettier feet from my doctor, I did fantasize prior to surgery about how much 'prettier'—those exact words—my feet might be, so I can understand why a woman having bunion surgery would ask her doctor to make her feet look prettier. When my surgery was complete and they removed the bandage, what I was most excited about wasn't the pain being over, but having a normal-looking foot and toe. This lasted all of six months. The curve returned and a slight bunion is forming again."

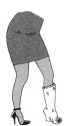

Scary Surgery Stories

READ THE gruesome details of what happened to these women, and you will appreciate your toes the way they are.

Patricia, age forty-four, from northern Virginia, had bunion and hammertoe surgery two years ago. Before the surgery, she had been a long-distance runner. Today, she can no longer run, has trouble walking, is in chronic pain, and has a deformed-looking foot.

"I don't like to talk about this. I just want to get past it. But if I can prevent just one woman from going through what I did, then it's worth it to talk about it.

"I was a long-distance runner. That was my outlet in life. But my left foot hurt me when I ran because I had a bunion. I had a bunion on my right foot also, but it didn't hurt yet, two years ago. I met with doctors who advised me against the surgery. They said I should give up running and wear supportive shoes and I would be fine. But I didn't want to hear that because I so much wanted to run. So I met with an orthopedic surgeon and I let myself get sucked in. He made me think he could fix the problem and I could continue running. He also claimed I had a hammertoe. I didn't think I had one—if I did, it was extremely mild—but he told me he could fix both at the same time. He downplayed how serious the surgery was. But he had a good reputation, and I looked him up and there were no complaints lodged against him.

"So I had the surgery. For the bunion, he told me during the consultation, he was going to put in screws, which would be removed a few weeks later, and for the hammertoe, he was to do the same thing but using pins. There wasn't supposed to be anything permanent left in my body. But the doctor told me that right after I was anesthetized he changed his mind and would use an implant, not pins, for the hammertoe.

"When the bandages came off it was tremendously painful. There was a rash with bumps all over my foot around the hammertoe incision. But the doctor dismissed me and cut me off when I asked about it. He told me that this was normal. So I went home, but the rash spread over my body and my foot swelled up. I went to his office and was told to sit in the waiting room. Finally he saw me and insisted that there was nothing wrong, even though it was obvious to everyone who saw me that there was something horribly wrong. So I went to the ER. The ER doctor said I had an allergic reaction or an infection but that he could not admit me to the hospital because my orthopedist had to admit me. So I went back to the orthopedist's office. By this point the rash had spread to my face. Once he saw my face all of a sudden, for the first time, he acted concerned, although he did not take responsibility. I ended up staying in the hospital for a week. Thank god I had insurance. I was on steroids, antibiotics, and an IV drip. I spent additional weeks seeing dermatologists.

"I was convinced that the implant was the culprit. The orthopedist refused to give me any information about it but I did research and discovered that it contained a small amount of nickel, which could have caused the problem. In the end he removed the implant, which had been inserted for a hammertoe that I never had a problem with in the first place. But he never removed the screws from the bunion area.

"I have chronic pain at the bunion area. It's worse than it was before the surgery. In the hammertoe area, I can't move my second toe at all because he removed all the tendons. It is short and warped-looking, although at this point I don't even care what it looks like. I can't run, and when I walk my gait is off because my second toe does not lie flat. The surgery was the stupidest thing I've ever done in my life."

Elyse Hoed, age twenty-three, underwent bunion surgery four years ago in Miami. Today, she continues to suffer from foot pain and can't wear most types of shoes.

"I was a cheerleader for eight years and started to experience foot pain in my left foot that would shoot up to my knee. I went to a podiatrist and learned that I had a bunion on my big toe and pinky toe. I was encouraged to have the surgery because I was young and I was told I would recover quickly. I was very cautious and met with different surgeons before deciding to go through with it. I finally chose an older doctor and younger doctor team. They told me that after the surgery my foot would be much more narrow, and that a lot of supermodels get this surgery in order to fit into certain shoes. For me that has been a complete contradiction since this surgery has limited the types of shoes I can wear.

"It has been four years, and my foot has yet to heal a hundred percent. During my college years I worked as a bartender, and I went home every night with a swollen foot, unable to bend my toes. Now I have a job that requires me to dress nicely. But I am unable to wear closed-toe, high-heel shoes because of the pressure on my foot. It swells when it's in a confined space for too long, and I often go home at the end of the day with a very swollen foot.

"The surgery was not botched, but it is a major surgery and it can have a negative outcome."

Bobbi Leder, from Houston, had bunion surgery when she was twenty. That was nineteen years ago. Her bunion returned almost immediately and she can't move her big toe.

"I developed genetic bunions at the age of eight. By the time I was twenty, I could barely walk in shoes since the bunion on my right foot had become so severe. The surgery was a necessity. Because I was under my mother's health insurance plan I didn't have many choices. I had to use the orthopedic surgeon in network near our house.

"The surgeon used lightweight pins to hold the bone after the procedure. While my foot was in the cast, one of the pins migrated deep into my foot. The doctor never took X-rays during the two months I wore the cast, so he had no idea. Without the pins, the bone went back to the way it was and the operation was for nothing. I had to have a second operation to remove the pins after the cast was removed. The pin-removal surgery was supposed to take a few minutes but wound up taking an hour because the pin that had migrated was embedded very deeply and the doctor couldn't find it.

"Then there was terrible inflammation. In nonmedical terms, the big toe was frozen and would not move when I walked. Fortunately, health insurance covered nine months of physical therapy. The therapist informed me that what I thought was inflammation was in fact the bunion. It was back, or never was fixed.

"Today I do not have full range of motion in my first metatarsal. My big toe is very stiff despite the physical therapy as well as toe exercises. I also have a long, thick keloid scar, and it's just as bad today as it was nineteen years ago. The scar actually hurts if it's touched. I also have scars where the pins were.

"The procedure was very painful, and it was a waste of time, money, and energy, not to mention that it caused the scar. I have since been to many podiatrists and they all agree that screws, not pins, should have been used. Live and learn. Today, my other foot hurts, and I've developed 'tailor's bunions' on both feet, but I will never put myself through another procedure like that again."

Betty Kerber, from Minnetonka, Minnesota, had hammertoe surgery when she was forty-two. Now fifty-six, she recently had to have two of her toes removed as a result of that procedure.

"I had hammertoes on all four small toes on my left foot. They weren't that bad and I shouldn't have had the surgery. The doctor inserted pins in toes 2 and 3, but never removed them. I didn't ask him about it because I thought he knew what he was doing. With toes 4 and 5, he removed the bones and fused them together.

"After the surgery, none of the four toes touched the floor. They all stuck up. The doctor said, 'But they aren't supposed to touch the floor!' That did not make sense to me. I went back to him again and said that something was not right, and that I wouldn't pay the balance of my bill until he corrected what was wrong. I requested my medical record, but he refused to give it to me since I hadn't completed the payment. Soon after, he was killed in a car accident. I never did get my record.

"I've been to several podiatrists over the years and they say they can't take out the pins now. Toes 2 and 3 are very rigid and can't bend or move. Toes 4 and 5 were just flaps of skin that would hang there. They were constantly getting infections and they retracted. So I had them removed. I only have three toes on my left foot now.

"My foot is always in pain. It is extremely sensitive. I have to wear padded shoes with support. It is too painful to be barefoot. It is also hard to keep my balance.

"My advice to someone thinking about foot surgery is to get at least three different opinions and to ask about complications."

DURING MY interview with her, Levine mostly played up the nonsurgical side of her spa. The Institute Beauté offers treatments such as bleaching of yellowed toenails, corn removal, Botox injections for the foot (to prevent the smell of excessive sweat), and a luxe pedicure called a "foot facial." (I complimented the playful name. "That was my term," she made sure I knew. "That is a trademarked term.") You can also come in for an array of expensive beauty treatments that have nothing to do with the foot—laser hair removal, wart removal, microdermabrasion, and Botox injections for the face.

Levine was most eager to talk about injecting cushioning material—marketed under the brand names Juvéderm and Sculptra—under the ball of the foot. She named this procedure "Pillows for Your Feet" (and again, trademarked the name). The theory is that the cushioning replaces the fat that age has eroded and thereby allows the wearing of high-heeled shoes. "That's been the most successful instead of doing surgery to change the structure of the foot. It is relatively conservative as far as I'm concerned. It enables women to wear shoes for a longer period of time. You leave the bunion as it is." The procedure must be repeated every six to nine months and starts at $500 per foot per treatment.

Levine's medical spa is also the site of an organization that she and Lautin co-launched in 2005 called the International Aesthetic Foot Society (IAFS). Levine and Lautin hold lectures and training sessions for members of the society, according to the society's website, teaching the "latest techniques for treating complications" and demonstrating how to do the ball-of-foot injections. They also offer marketing tips on "How To Get Press for Your Practice." A podiatrist from South Miami, Dr. Cynthia Marzouka-Losito, has been featured on the IAFS website because she took Levine and Lautin's training session in 2007 and now injects Sculptra into feet for $1000 per foot.[38]

How does the medical community feel about "Pillows for Your Feet"? Injecting cushioning into the ball of the foot "is a ridiculous thing to do," according to Dreeben. "First, there is no correlation between the thickness of the foot pad and pain. Second, the material will degenerate or cause scarring. No matter what the material is, it won't hold up. Third, there can be enormous problems. Some people are allergic to these substances and develop huge granulomas, which are abnormal masses in the foot caused by your body reacting to a foreign substance. Sometimes the substance migrates and you can get nerve entrapment. I am appalled and surprised that this procedure is being done."

"Injections in the forefoot for cushioning is usually not good in the long term and even disastrous for someone who walks for extended periods of time," agrees Positano. "I have seen numerous women and men who have developed very painful scar tissue built up in the areas of these injections. There also can be nerve inflammation and damage. My advice is to pass on this. It is far safer and efficacious to have a prescription foot orthotic made to redistribute and decrease the force in the front of the feet."

But the woman looking for a quick fix so that she can wear the new peep-toe platforms does not want to be told to wear a sensible shoe with an orthotic instead. That is the whole point of the cosmetic foot surgery industry in the first place. "The way we've gone about trying to educate women is wrong," sighs Dreeben. Women don't listen when their doctor tells them to stop wearing heels, she says. "If *I* wear them, I can't tell other women not to wear them. So I use myself as a role model. I wear cute shoes to my office that my patients see me walking around in. I have a pair of leopard-print flats and other fashionable shoes that are comfortable. I tell my patients to have some fashionable, comfortable flats to wear during the day, and then bring their stilettos to dinner when they're just sitting down and not walking.

"I also make a point of showing my patients the insides of my shoes. I put in special pads for arch support. If I wear pointy-toe shoes, I buy them a half-size larger and put tissue inside the end of the toes. There are all these little tricks you can do. If you have a bunion or a bunionette, you bring your shoes to the repairman and have him stretch them out. I want my patients to see what we can do to alter our shoes. I tell them, 'I'm as vain as you are. If I can do it, you can do it.'"

The best of Youner's advice? She tells her patients, "If your feet are ugly, put on some pretty nail polish."

But What If You Need Surgery Because You're In Pain?

You've done everything you can to prevent bunion or hammertoe surgery. You've been wearing orthotics and wide-toed shoes; you've been exercising your toes; and you've been regularly checking in with your foot doctor. But now the pain is too intense and you believe that you have no alternative but to have surgery. What next? Register with the excellent blog BunionSurvivor.com, which is filled with sound advice. BunionSurvivor.com founder Mary Marcdante offers these suggestions:

- Do research on the Internet on the various types of surgery so that when you talk to your surgeon, you understand him or her.
- Ask at least five people who have already had the surgery which doctors they recommend or do not recommend.
- Get at least three opinions from both podiatrists and orthopedic foot surgeons.
- Ask lots of questions about what to expect and what Plan B is if the surgery doesn't work.
- Ask how many times the surgeon had to do additional surgery to correct problems for the first surgery.
- Listen to your intuition. If you don't feel comfortable with a surgeon's responses, find another doctor.

Chapter 5

THE HISTORY OF HIGH HEELS

WE LIVE in a sex-saturated culture where many women flaunt their sexuality freely. Female sexual exhibitionism is everywhere, from *Girls Gone Wild* videos to pole-dancing exercise classes to Brazilian waxes. Even little girls are made conscious of themselves as potentially sexual. They attend makeover parties at spas and wear thong underwear. No one raises an eyebrow when adult women wear skin-baring, curve-hugging, bra-strap-revealing attire. It's not even shocking to see fetish-themed corsets, leather, and rubber incorporated into women's fashions.

What has caused this new exhibitionist sexual ethic? There are myriad sources. Many girls and women confuse male attention with genuine power, believing that female sexual power is the only real power they possess. As author Erica Jong has said, "Sexual freedom can be a smokescreen for how far we *haven't* come."[39] We live in a culture with a deeply entrenched sexual double standard, in which girls and young women risk being considered "sluts" no matter what they do sexually. With these circumstances, why *not* take off your clothes—what do you have to lose? Since comprehensive sex education isn't widely available, young people of both sexes are left ignorant of what healthy sexuality looks like. And as queer sexuality becomes more open yet paradoxically remains stigmatized, there is increasing anxiety among heterosexuals to assert their straight credentials.

"It used to be that people said, 'You look pretty' or 'You look beautiful,'" observes Elizabeth Semmelhack, chief curator of the Bata Shoe Museum in Toronto. "Now it's 'You look hot' or 'You look sexy.'" If looking attractive is equated with looking sexy, then according to this logic the most flattering shoes are the sexiest ones. Women may tell themselves they're wearing high heels to look thinner or lovelier than they imagine themselves to be in one-inch wedges, but the idea of being thin and lovely is now inextricably associated with sex appeal. Whether consciously real-

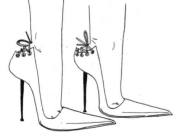

ized or not, women wear high heels to look sexy. What we wear on our feet is a big part of how we signify gender, class, race, and declare our personalities. Hippies wear Birkenstocks, punks wear combat boots, the cool kids wear the latest pair of sneakers, and sexy ladies wear sexy shoes.

In this environment women's shoes have increasingly come to resemble pornographic footwear. If you go to a department store, you will find "stripper platform shoes and dominatrix boots," observes Semmelhack. "These became very popular in the last ten years at the same time that normal underwear became replaced with stripper clothes, when camisoles became acceptable as outerwear. Clothing and shoes have become connected with sex work."

I ask Semmelhack about the increased popularity of flip-flops—how are they sexualized? "They are a signifier of leisure, and in our culture leisure is often connected with being in a state of undress," she points out. Seen from this perspective, the nakedness of the foot in a flip-flop is sexy too. Also, just as high heels signify wealth and status—since you can't do physical labor or go very far in them without a car—so too do flip-flops connote wealth and leisure. Semmelhack adds that when you wear flip-flops or any type of sandal, this "creates another level of necessary consumption—pedicures and nail polish. It adds this extra level of work you have to do to make yourself presentable. If you have leisure then you have the time to get your pedicure done." When women choose heels or flip-flops or other very revealing sandals when they are far from a pool or beach, they are asserting their identity as sexual and feminine women.

It has always been this way. Shoes have been regarded as a sexual prop for centuries. In fact, prostitutes have long been at the vanguard of footwear fashion. Through the centuries, ordinary women have followed the lead of "fallen women" in wearing erotically charged shoes. Men, too, have worn shoes with obvious sexual meaning. For both sexes, wearing these types of shoes has been a way to indicate one's sexual sophistication without risking social embarrassment. Clothing that is considered "too" revealing or "too" tight may be interpreted as a sign of sexual desperation, and therefore can be socially risky. But feet are not the focal point when we look at another person, opening up the opportunity to clothe the feet in riskier fashion. Sexually suggestive shoes, then, are often considered safer and more socially acceptable than sexually suggestive clothing.

In her engrossing book *Heights of Fashion: A History of the Elevated Shoe*, Semmelhack traced the story of how we got to the point where hardware-studded stilettos are acceptable in many offices.[40] It started in antiquity, when Greek, Etruscan, and Roman women wore platform shoes. After the fall of the Roman Empire, however, elevated shoes were abandoned by Western women, and did not reappear in the West for roughly another thousand years. (If you think waiting for coveted shoes from a designer's waiting list is hard, try a millennium.) Before and after the fall of Constantinople in 1453, refugees from the Ottoman Empire flooded Europe and introduced their new neighbors to the platform clog known as the *qabqab*, which kept feet dry while in public bathhouses. Wooden clogs on stilts soon became popular among upper-class men and women in Europe.

Between 1300 and 1500, a bizarre type of shoe with long, pointed toes was enormously popular with men. It was called a *poulaine* (meaning Poland) or a *crakow* (after the Polish city). "A normal set of toes would literally have needed to be scrunched one on top of the other," noted Colin McDowell in his book *Shoes: Fashion and Fantasy*.[41] The sexual symbolism was pronounced: the long toe was phallic. In some styles it was padded with horse hair and curled at the tip, and often the toes were three times as long as the foot. In these extreme styles it was impossible to walk, so men attached a string or wire between the tip of the shoe and their leg.

This did not sit well with clergymen. In 1468, a papal bull (a document issued by the pope) condemned the *poulaine* as "a scoffing against God and the church, a worldyly vanity and a mad presumption."[42] The bull tried to limit the length of the toe, but men paid no attention to it. One fifteenth-century Italian preacher denounced the shoes on the grounds that the shape showed a lack of respect for Jesus Christ, whose feet had been nailed to the cross for the sake of mankind. Interestingly, the shoes themselves were uncomfortable and created a feeling of "martyring" the feet for the sake of fashion.[43]

Meanwhile, women wanted elevated shoes of their own. Shoemakers in fifteenth-century Italy and Spain complied and created an eroticized, womanly platform shoe known in Venice as the *chopine* (pronounced: sho-PEEN). The height of *chopines* puts today's heels to shame. Eleven-inch platforms were not unusual, and the tallest surviving pair is twenty inches tall. It was impossible to walk in *chopines* without someone, or even two people, assisting the wearer. Originally they were

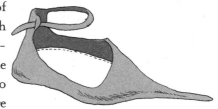

created to keep one's feet out of the dirt and mud on the streets, but Venetian courtesans adopted an extravagant form of *chopine* as their trademark. This development made it scandalous for "respectable" women to wear them; but we have evidence that women across the social spectrum did just that anyway. It was impossible to miss the sexual overtones. Not only were these shoes worn by prostitutes; they were also eroticized because they so obviously restricted a woman's mobility. *Chopines* were highly coveted and frequently represented in paintings, frescoes, and prints. In many cities in Italy preachers condemned these shoes, citing Matthew 6:27, a verse understood to prohibit the increasing of one's height.[44] "Sumptuary laws"—which regulated dress—limited the height of women's shoes. Women who broke the law were forced to pay a fine.

Cobblers could not keep up with the demand. Beginning in the 1500s and continuing until the 1880s, they were forced to cut down on one of the time-consuming tasks that prevented them from producing enough pairs. Instead of creating shoes to fit a left foot and a right foot, they began making soles that could fit either foot, with no distinction

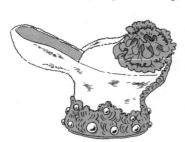

between the two, called "straights." This practice meshed with a desire for symmetry. Since other dual parts of the body (eyes, legs, arms, and so on) appear symmetrical, it made sense that feet should too.[45] We can assume that between the straight shape and the extreme height, shoes of this period were pretty uncomfortable to wear.

The high heel wasn't introduced to Western Europe until the late sixteenth century. Some historians claim that the heel was simply a modification of the *chopine,* but Semmelhack argues otherwise. Men, not women, wore heels first, and Semmelhack claims that there is no way upper-class men would have taken for themselves, however transformed, something so heavily associated with sexualized femininity. More likely, they tweaked Persian male equestrian and military footwear to fit their needs. The heel was functional because it kept a rider's feet planted firmly in stirrups. It was considered exotic and a sign of adventure because it had an Eastern tinge. Its equestrian and military roots also evoked sexual virility. Soon enough men realized that their high-heeled shoes needed some further fine-tuning to enable them to go out into the public with ease. Their shoes became sturdier and more durable; they could withstand the outdoors.

Upper-class European women followed in men's footsteps and abandoned the *chopine* for the heeled shoe. Unlike men's high-heeled shoes, theirs were delicate and refined—appropriate only for the indoors. Gendered differences in heeled footwear were evident during the period of Louis XIV, king of France from 1643 to 1715. Louis XIV is well known for his opulence and decadence—and for being five foot five. He wore shoes with heels that were decorated with elaborate miniature paintings of battles or landscapes. He declared that only those aristocrats who were part of his court were permitted to wear shoes with red heels—instantly transforming shoes with red heels into coveted signs of privilege and access. But the heels he and other aristocratic men wore were not feminized. By and large their shoes were squared off at the toes, had heels moderate in height, and were decorated with a buckle. Their shoes connoted strength. Interestingly, a decoration known as the "shoe rose" became popular, but this large silk pompon on the front of the shoe was considered masculine because it served as a phallic symbol.[46]

Women, on the other hand, wore heels that were narrower and higher. The toe box was pointed and the shoes were decorated with ribbon laces and other feminine accoutrements. Their shoes were created to make the foot appear smaller than it actually was. Women today often pair high heels with long pants that hide most of the shoe and expose only the toes. Similarly, back in the days of the French aristocracy, wrote Semmelhack, women "gave the impression of a tiny foot by hiding the greater part of the foot under the skirt and revealing just the enticing tip of the shoe at the hemline."[47]

The upper classes wore heels for status. When the lower classes began to wear high-heeled shoes, the affluent had to figure out how to distinguish themselves. Their solution was to raise the height of the heel—the higher the heel, the more impractical the shoe, the higher the class status. But very high heels were not meant for outdoor wear. After all, the roads were unpaved. Heels would sink into the muck. What were status-conscious members of the gentry to do? First they experimented with a flat-soled mule that worked like an overshoe. When they went outside, they would simply slip

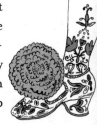

on the overshoe. Before long, high-heeled shoes became integrated into the flat-soled mule in a contraption called the "slap sole" (so called because the sole made a slapping sound when the wearer walked in them). Alternately, a *patten*—an iron ring attached to the bottom of the shoe—enabled the wearer to venture outside without ruining his or her heels.

Enlightenment ideas about reason, freedom, and democracy began to brew in Europe. The allure of the aristocracy was on the wane. Men abandoned the high heel and other ostentatious displays. Except for a blip in the 1970s when platforms became stylish for men as well as women, elevated shoes from this point on were a women-only affair. Women continued to wear high heels, and this practice was offered up as evidence that only men were capable of being enlightened, rational beings. After all, high heels were ludicrously impractical. Semmelhack cites a popular French ditty from this period:

> "Mount on French heels
> When you go to a ball
> 'Tis the fashion to totter
> And show you can fall."[48]

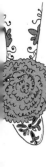

Surely women were not as rational as men if they chose fashion slavery over the freedom of enfranchisement. In 1792, the British feminist Mary Wollstonecraft warned that girls who were denied education and socialized to care only about fashion were growing up to live in a "gilt cage."[49]

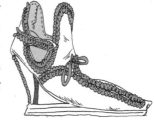

After the American and French revolutions, most women came to agree that the high heel was not in step with contemporary values, and chose flat-soled shoes instead. This trend dovetailed with nineteenth-century beliefs about womanhood. The best woman, it was now maintained, was a domestic mother whose primary role was providing a moral education for her children. Flat shoes enabled mothers to live a hectic life attending to children's needs.

But as we know, fashion is cyclical. By the middle of the nineteenth century, women of privilege began wearing close-fitting, high-buttoned boots with a heel again. In her 1831 autobiography, the French novelist George Sand compared the experience of wearing women's shoes with wearing men's shoes.

"On the Paris pavement I was like a boat on ice. My delicate shoes cracked open in two days, my pattens had me spinning, and I always forgot to lift my dress. I was muddy . . . and I watched my shoes and my clothes . . . go to rack and ruin with alarming rapidity. . . . [To save money, I began to dress as a young man.] I can't convey how much my boots delighted me: I'd have gladly slept in them, as my brother did when he was a lad and had just got his first pair. With those steel-tipped heels I was solid on the sidewalk at last. I dashed back and forth across Paris and felt I was going around the world."[50]

Meanwhile, African-American slaves were forced to wear stiff, shoddy shoes called "brogans." These shoes had thick wooden or leather soles. They were constructed by unskilled, poorly paid laborers who received low wages compared with other shoemakers. After the Emancipation Proclamation and the Thirteenth Amendment, which abolished slavery, shoemakers reported that no one wanted to buy brogans anymore because they had become so indelibly associated with forced and degrading servitude.[51]

By the end of the nineteenth century, urban renewal led to the creation of department stores in Paris, London, and New York. The industrialization of shoemaking meant that one no longer had to visit a shoemaker and have her feet measured to order a pair of shoes. Now there was an array of readymade, mass-manufactured, fashionable shoes from which to choose. Women in Europe and the United States were more mobile and independent than they had ever been before, and those who could spent their leisure time walking on the streets, visiting cafés, and shopping for pleasure.

You might conclude that this mobility motivated them to choose practical shoes meant for walking. But you would be wrong. The opposite occurred: now that women were in public and on display, they felt it was more important than ever before to wear feminine, high-heeled shoes. Before, "respectable" women had been pressured to stay at home and protect the domestic haven, and only prostitutes or "fallen" women had ventured outside on a regular basis. But now women across the social spectrum were strutting around independently, conspicuously, and erotically. No matter how much their preachers warned that heels were improper, women refused to give them up.

It was now commonly known that high-heeled shoes caused pain to the wearer, not only in the feet but also in the knees and back. Some women experiencing pain could limit the number of hours they wore high-heeled shoes, but the women working in department stores and clothing stores were pressured to wear the items they sold—and these women were on their feet for twelve to fourteen hours a day. In 1880, the British medical journal the *Lancet* editorialized against this "cruelty to women," and physicians in Paris, London, and New York attempted to enact legislation requiring employers to provide seats for female employees so that they wouldn't be forced to stand in heels all day.[52]

By the beginning of the twentieth century, high heels were ubiquitous in the United States. Even suffragists, accused of being unattractive and unfeminine and therefore irrelevant (as women's rights advocates always have been), wore them. "The women who desire votes are paying more attention to their appearance," the *New York Times* reported triumphantly in 1912. The *Times* quoted a suffragist who had said, "They are now recognizing the fact that for women to appear untidy or weirdly dressed in unfashionable garments . . . damages the cause for which they are working."[53] But when it comes to feminine attire, you can never win no matter what you wear. Other suffragists attacked their high-heel-shod sisters: "I beg to advance the following thesis: The efficient life cannot be lived on French heels."[54] In 1908, *Ladies' Home Journal* published X-rays of a foot in high heels and low heels to demonstrate that "the bones of the foot are forced into an unnatural relation to each other."[55] Women who continued to wear heels had been warned.

If there had been any uneasiness about the erotic associations of the high heel, they were laid aside after the deaths of millions of men during World War I and the flu pandemic of 1918 to 1920. Women wanted to look as sexually alluring as possible to compete for the few remaining marriageable men, and those who were most daring took up the "flapper" fashion—no corset, high hemline, heavy makeup, and high heels. Flappers were audaciously sexual in their appearance. The majority of American women had no interest in adopting the flapper ensemble in its entirety, but one item was popular across the board: high heels.

Because of the high heel's sexual suggestiveness, which was seen as immoral, high schools and colleges threatened to prohibit them, and state legislatures introduced bills banning them. And mingled with religious and moral denunciations were health warnings. In 1920, the *Washington Post* reported on the speech of a well-known surgeon. "Animated with a holy zeal for *the preservation of both health and morality,* he denounced the vile thing in every mood and tense," the reporter observed. "The distinguished surgeon went on to record as being wishful to send to the penitentiary all manufacturers of high heels on the ground of mayhem and mutilation" [italics mine].[56] It is unfortunate that the very legitimate health claims against high heels were invoked in the same breath as tenuous arguments about immorality. Perhaps had the health warnings been isolated as a singular deficiency of high-heeled footwear, women would have listened more closely.

After the stock market crash of 1929, a subdued look in women's clothing and shoes became the standard. Unemployment and underemployment meant more free time and less money, so Americans sought leisure-time activities that were free, like going to the beach. Open-toed sandals became popular as a result, and Italian shoe designer Salvatore Ferragamo transformed the beach sandal into chic wedge heels and platform sandals. Women far from sand and seaweed wore the wedge and the platform, which were considered fashionable but not sexual.

During World War II, women continued to wear the wedge and the platform; they were more sensible than heels but nevertheless feminine and attractive. Women became concerned not only with their shoes' design but with the practical issue of their fit. A 1945 magazine ad by Gold Cross Shoes promised:

"You can't buy a new Gold Cross Shoe style until it's Fit-Tested for weeks on active, human feet. Before any Gold Cross style is introduced, handmade originals are worn . . . walked in . . . for weeks. Checked, daily, by our designers for even a hint of gapping, wrinkling, binding. Changed. Checked again. Until the kind of fit is assured that millions of women tell you they find *only* in . . . America's famous Fit-Tested footwear."[57]

During the war, women's shoes matched their sober, masculinized clothes: knee-length skirts paired with long jackets. The millions of women working in factories, assisting the war effort and covering for the men who were overseas, by necessity wore practical lace-up shoes during the day. But when they weren't in grimy factories, they continued to wear stylish, though de-eroticized, fashions.

The men fighting overseas, however, were simultaneously exposed to a very different image of femininity: the "pinup" or scantily attired voluptuous model in high heels. Posters and postcards of sexy pinups provided soldiers with an idealized image to dream about, which boosted their morale during excruciatingly frightening and horrible wartime conditions. When the men came home, many were disappointed that their real wives and girlfriends did not measure up to their beloved pinups. Let's face it: who could? But countless women tried their hardest. They shoved their wedges and platforms to the back of the closet and went out to purchase sexy high heels. Since their wartime jobs were wrested from them and handed back to the boys, they didn't see a need for sensible shoes any longer anyway.

The Doctors Warned, and Warned, and Warned

In every generation, medical professionals have cautioned women that high heels are bad news.

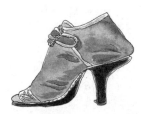

1740

"Not only the muscles of the large Achilles tendon which serve the extension of the foot, but also the anterior muscles which serve the extension of the toes, are as a result of the height of these shoes continually in a state of forced contraction; and not only the anterior muscles which serve the flexion of the foot, but the posterior muscles which serve the flexion of the toes, are at the same time as a result of this height continually in a state of forced elongation. This continual state of contraction of some and of tugging of the others of these muscles can only cause sooner or later some more or less considerable harm to their vessels, both blood and lymphatic, and to their nerves, and moreover by means of the communication of these vessels and of these nerves with the vessels and the nerves of other more distant parts, even with those of the viscera of the abdomen, etc., occasion discomforts that one would attribute to a totally different cause, and consequently one would continually bring to bear remedies not only useless but accidentally harmful and dangerous."[58]

—Jacob Winslow, professor of anatomy, Jardin du Roi, Paris

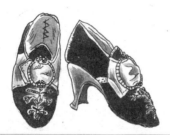

1781

"The wealthy women walk . . . by reason of the height of their heels, on the fore-ends of their feet, and consequently, very badly; they walk, if it is permitted to make this comparison, like the majority of quadrupeds—on their toes only."[59]

—Peter Camper, chair of anatomy and surgery, Athenaeum, Amsterdam

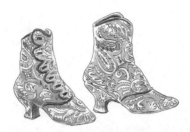

1868

"High-heeled boots and shoes are universal, notwith-standing that medical men have been writing very severely against them. They say that the fashion causes corns, cramps, lameness at an early age, lessens the size of the calf, and thus makes the leg lose its symmetry."[60]
—British women's magazine

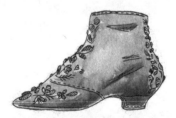

1882

"I have heard a story that a lady who had been wearing these high-heeled shoes went to one of the most celebrated orthopedic surgeons in New York City for some spinal trouble, and when, after examining the case, he found that she was wearing a pair of these fashionable shoes, he immediately seized them and with language more forcible than elegant pulled off the heels and flung them away, following them with a shower of denunciations, and prophesying all sorts of ill results should the abominable fashion be continued."[61]

—Fordyce Barker, president of the New York Academy of Medicine

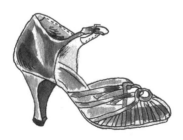

1934

"High-heeled shoes, if worn for long periods, lead to serious changes in body mechanics and in the alignment of the foot."[62]

—Popular medical textbook

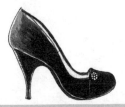

1952

"Excessively high heels will always be a source of danger to feet and eventually to health. Their habitual use causes the calf muscles to contract to such an extent that . . . it becomes almost impossible to walk either barefoot or in slippers. . . . Thick ankles and mildly deformed feet are among the direct products of shoes with six-inch heels."[63]
—George Bankoff, British surgeon

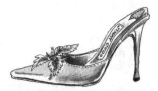

2000

"Compared with males, females have 9:1 odds of having various forefoot problems develop. It can be concluded that males wear more 'healthy' shoes. Shoes for males provide a roomier, nonconstricting environment for the foot than fashion shoes for females. The orthopaedist might conclude that women would wear roomier shoes if they were informed of the ill-effects of wearing constricting shoewear. Unfortunately, this is often not the case. Women's high fashion shoes are extremely popular, not because women are illogical in their selection of shoewear, but because the selection of women's high fashion shoes is a part of a much larger pattern of human behavior in which people who alter their appearance become more appealing socially and sexually."[64]

—Carol Frey, clinical assistant professor of orthopaedic surgery, UCLA

IN THE history of high heels, things started to get particularly interesting after the war ended. In films noir of 1946—*The Postman Always Rings Twice* with Lana Turner and *Double Indemnity* with Barbara Stanwyck—the camera lingers on closeup shots of the heels of the femme fatales. The audience knows that these women are dangerous because of their seductive shoes. High-heeled shoes mean that a woman is dressed to kill.

In 1947, Christian Dior introduced a curvaceous, hourglass silhouette with a cinched waist, fitted bust, padded hips, and crinolined skirt. Called the "New Look," Dior's clothing had a tremendous impact on the world of fashion because it was, in effect, an announcement that it was time for women to start dressing like sexual beings again. But a "new look" always requires new shoes to punctuate the silhouette. Dior's look necessitated an elegant high heel to complete it.

The prevailing wisdom, then and now, is that high heels look sexiest when the heel is very narrow. Shoe designers attempted to create high-heeled shoes with narrow heels but were stymied because of limited technology. In the 1940s, heels had been made of wood and covered with leather. If the heel tapered too much, it could not support the weight of the woman wearing it without snapping.[65] In the 1950s, shoe manufacturers in Italy solved the problem of how to create an ultra-narrow high heel. They inserted a metal rod enclosed in a plastic heel shell. The metal rod supported the weight of the woman wearing the shoe and enabled heels to elevate to five inches.

In 1952, Roger Vivier, Dior's shoe designer, created the classic pump. It had a four-inch tapered heel with a pointed toe. Other designers, such as Charles Jourdan, Herman Delman, and Salvatore Ferragamo, likewise tapered their high heels. *Vogue* magazine described these shoes as "stiletto"—meaning "little knife" in Italian.

It's hard to ignore the violent meaning of a shoe called a "little knife." Perhaps women eagerly adopted the stiletto as a way to passively express their anger about having been forced out of their wartime employment. Or, perhaps the stiletto was a symbol of refusal to do housework; as shoe historian Caroline Cox suggested, it could be understood as "a sign of open resistance, a challenge to male-dominated culture by wearing shoes that quite clearly signaled, 'I haven't tidied up today.'"[66]

But in fact, many women did tidy up while wearing high heels. They felt pressured to strive to resemble pinups or other glamorous, famous, sexually alluring women *all the time.* Marilyn Monroe wiggled her behind in stilettos, and *Playboy,* inaugurated in 1953, showcased "girls next door" who were naked but for their stilettos. These highly eroticized shoes became normative footwear, even while doing chores inside the home.

In the early 1960s, the toe box of the stiletto was narrowed into an exaggeratedly elongated point that recalled the *poulaines* of the fifteenth century. This new style, called the "winklepicker" (the name of a tool used to extract snails from their shells) was wildly popular in Britain among both males and females. "Aesthetically, the combination of the sharp-pointed toe and stiletto heel provided the perfect complement to the foot, ankle, and calf," wrote shoe historian Jonathan Walford, "but from a medical viewpoint it was a terrible mix."[67] In 1971, Abigail Van Buren, also known as "Dear Abby," sent an open letter to the National Shoe Manufacturers' Association, along with a hundred thousand letters of support from American women. She wrote, "Please do what you can, when

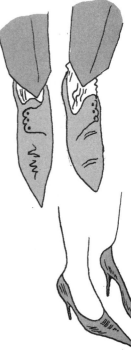

you can, gentlemen, to liberate the captive feet of womanhood. It's not fair and it's not fun to hurt from the ground up in the name of fashion."[68] If no one cared about the permanent physical damage women were doing to their feet, they did become alarmed about the destruction of wooden floors. Throughout the 1960s, museums, galleries, and historic sites banned the stiletto to protect their flooring.

High heels went on the decline for a few years in the 1960s. In the middle of the decade, the premier fashion model was Twiggy, who affected a "lost little girl" appearance with miniskirts, tights, and low-heeled shoes and André Courrèges go-go boots. Millions of stylish women copied her look. This trend, coupled a few years later with the women's liberation arguments against high heels, girdles, and garter belts, made stilettos unfashionable. In the 1970s, the clunky platform shoe reappeared, and even men wore them during this period of androgyny. Shoes with contoured foot beds, such as Birkenstock sandals and "negative-heeled shoes" (in which the heel sits lower than the toes), also became available in the 1970s, appealing to those who had chosen to stand outside of fashion in the name of comfort and health.

In the 1980s, an increasing number of women entered the workforce. Unsure of what to wear to look professional, millions took the advice of John T. Molloy, a wardrobe consultant and author of *The Woman's Dress for Success Book*, who advised them to wear a dark-colored conservative skirt suit with medium-height heels. "The best shoe for a businesswoman is the plain pump, in a dark color, with closed toe and heel," Molloy wrote. "The heel should be about an inch and a half." Molloy argued that when a man wears a suit and tie it is as if he is wearing a sign that says "Businessman." Women need the same sign. The dark skirted suit and pump combination, he promised, "will give businesswomen a look of authority, which is precisely what they need. If women are to enjoy widespread success in all industries, they must adopt this uniform. It is their best hope."[69] Molloy believed that this uniform would make career women appear serious, modest, professional, but feminine at the same time.

In his best-selling book, Molloy attacked the fashion industry for offering women clothes that were too erotic or too domestic for them to be taken as seriously as men. He warned women who wanted to succeed in business to ignore fashion trends. It is not surprising, then, that the fashion industry largely ignored Molloy's message. Clothing and shoe manufacturers never want to sell women a basic conservative uniform because it's in their financial interest to sell new silhouettes and designs each season. "Power dressing" in the eyes of the fashion industry ended up looking corporate only from the waist up: the uniform became a jacket with broad shoulders paired with a short skirt and stilettos. But most career women shrewdly saved their stilettos for after work, choosing medium-height heels for the office. They recognized that if they wore overtly eroticized shoes during the day, they would not have been taken seriously as professionals.

That viewpoint seems perfectly quaint by today's fashion standards.

In the twenty-first century, women in many industries wear sexually suggestive shoes to work every day. "Toe cleavage," the exposure of a hint of a woman's toes when her shoe is cut low in the toe box, is commonplace and acceptable in many corporate offices (while breast cleavage is not). With each season, heels become narrower and more pointed at the toe, looking increasingly like the exaggerated "winklepickers" of the early 1960s.

In 2003, designer Manolo Blahnik announced that his new line of shoes would be 20 percent narrower and more pointed than in previous seasons, which seemed utterly impossible at the time given how narrow and pointed they already were.[70] In the summer of 2009, bondage- and fetish-themed shoes were featured in all nonorthopedic shoe stores. Nine West sold a sandal that was typical of the season: four-inch heel, studded leather overlapping straps, with "rear zip entry" (according to the company's website). This style, the Kentaro, was called a "cheap thrill" by *Women's Wear Daily*.[71]

If we look at history, we see that this cycle won't last forever. But it is possible that it could go on for a while. "If the current spike-heel madness continues," wrote Simon Doonan, creative director of Barneys New York, "I fear that my old age is doomed to be spent pushing all my chums around in wheelchairs." Doonan added an irreverent PS: there is one good thing about sitting in a wheelchair, he noted—you can wear "really insanely pornographic" shoes without hurting yourself.[72]

Chapter 6

THE SEX LIFE OF WOMEN'S SHOES

SOMETIMES A shoe is not just a shoe: it is a stand-in for something else.

In the Hebrew Bible, shoes are removed a number of times and very often this act suggests a heightened level of intimacy, either between a human and God or between two people. The most famous shoe-removal incident is when Moses approaches the presence of God at the burning bush. God tells Moses to remove his shoes because the ground is holy. [73] Standing in the harsh desert without the protection of his shoes, Moses is vulnerable and, in a spiritual sense, naked before God. A ritual described in Deuteronomy allows a man to refuse to marry his deceased brother's widow (whom he would otherwise be obligated to wed). The widow removes her brother-in-law's sandal, spits in his face, and denounces him. [74] It has been suggested that this "unshoeing" was a form of "symbolic emasculation." [75] In commenting on the Bible, the great rabbis living in Babylonia from 200 to 600 CE used the word "shoe" as a euphemism for a vagina and also, in other contexts, for a penis.[76]

To be sure, shoes do not always symbolize intimacy or sexuality. In biblical and folkloric texts, shoes have also been used to formalize legal transactions, as a sign of the spirit of the person who wore them, and as a mark of dominance. Nevertheless, there are many customs across cultures involving shoes that hint at sexual meaning. Brides and grooms throughout history and in different parts of the world have been given shoes as wedding gifts and have been pelted with slippers as they have departed on their honeymoon, with members of the community saying to the groom, "May you fit her as well as my foot fits this old shoe."[77] In Bedouin divorce, the husband declares, "She is my slipper, I have cast her off."[78] In some parts of China, it is traditional for a woman trying to conceive to take a shoe from the temple of the god-

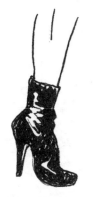

dess who has the power to bring children. When the child arrives, the mother returns the shoe to the goddess.

When its eroticism is taken to an extreme degree, the shoe can become a fetish object. Most of us associate the word ""fetish" exclusively with sadomasochistic or uncommon sexual preferences. But "fetish" means simply an object mistakenly believed to have supernatural power. It was originally used to

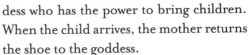

describe idol worship since only God, not an idol, is supposed to be all-powerful. (One could make the case that God worship is also fetishistic, in which case idol worship is just the replacement of one fetish for another.) In the nineteenth century, Karl Marx cheekily appropriated the term in his development of the concept of "commodity fetishism"—the mistaken belief that commodities have inherent value, which erases the value of the labor of people who produce the commodities. Later in the century, the psychologist Alfred Binet used "fetish" in a sexual sense. The 1870 novel *Venus in Furs* by Leopold von Sacher-Masoch explores the world of sexual fetishes, as well as domination and submission, prompting the psychiatrist Richard Freiherr von Krafft-Ebing to coin the term "masochism." (We can also thank Krafft-Ebing for "sadism," named after the Marquis de Sade.)

But it was the psychoanalyst Sigmund Freud who most successfully sharpened the concept of sexual fetishism. According to Freud, a fetish object develops when a young boy (always a boy, never a girl) sees that his mother lacks a penis. This is a terrifying discovery because he believes that his mother has been castrated—and if his all-powerful mother could be castrated, then so could he, a mere little boy. The boy fixates on his mother's foot or shoe, the last thing his eyes glimpsed before he looked up and met the horrible reality of her "missing" penis. The foot or shoe in turn becomes a symbolic substitute for the "missing" penis. (The fetish object is not necessarily a foot or shoe, but these are the most common symbolic substitutes.) The boy later forgets this transformative moment but forever associates erotic desire with the fetish object, which enables him to grow up and engage in heterosexual relations without anxiety. In the boy's mind, Freud writes,

"[T]he woman *has* got a penis, in spite of everything; but this penis is no longer the same as it was before. Something else has taken its place, has been appointed its substitute, as it were, and now inherits the interest which was formerly directed to its predecessor. But this interest suffers an extraordinary increase as well, because the horror of castration has set up a memorial to itself in the creation of this substitute. . . . [The fetish] remains a token of triumph over the threat of castration and a protection against it."[79]

As Freud describes it, this specific scenario of a boy fixing on the image of his mother's foot or shoe as he looks up her dress and discovers her vulva seems absurd. Are we really supposed to believe that every man with a foot or shoe fetish (there are more of them than you may imagine) underwent this precise process of discovery, terror, and denial? But we can accept Freud's concept of the sexual fetish object without taking his fantastical scene as literal truth. The important point Freud makes is that the woman's foot or shoe becomes a symbol of her genitals. For many men, this fetish enables them to engage in a healthy sexual life, although for others the fetish object takes the place of a sex partner and becomes an obstacle to a satisfying sexual life.

The English psychoanalyst John C. Flügel took Freud's model one step further. He argued that a woman's shoe is actually "ambisexual" because it can represent *both* the female genitals *and* the penis.[80] Flügel's theory makes sense: if the foot is reminiscent of the penis, then the shoe would correspondingly symbolize the vagina, since a foot entering into the opening of a tight-fitting, delicate shoe is reminiscent of coitus. Alternately, the shoe itself can appear phallic if it has a high heel and/or a pointy toe, studs, or bondage-inspired leather straps.

But what about *women* with a shoe fetish? Some girls and women do experience penis envy and unconsciously believe that they are supposed to have a penis but that it is missing. On an unconscious level, they believe that their body is wounded or damaged. This leads to feelings of inferiority and, for some, lifelong attempts to overcome these feelings. For these women, wearing phallic shoes can be a method of compensation. But drawing from the work of the French psychoanalyst Jacques Lacan, a number of feminist psychoanalysts, such as Judith Butler and Teresa de Lauretis, have theorized that women go through a different process. In this scenario, a woman feels a profound sense of loss not connected with the phallus at all but rather over closeness with her mother's body. As a young girl, she experiences an intense tactile relationship with her mother but as she becomes older and separated from her mother, this physical closeness disintegrates. Wearing shoes that remind her of her mother—and, as we have seen, a woman's shoe can symbolize the vagina—is a way to address feelings of sadness over the necessary but painful separation. These melancholy feelings of loss connected with separation can also be experienced by men.

Many shoe lovers, though not necessarily sexually risqué in the bedroom, in fact do think about women's shoes in fetishistic ways. How so? First, as we have seen in Chapter 2, many women ascribe a sense of intrinsic transformative power to their shoes that does not make rational sense for a protective article of clothing. Second, women's shoes that are not eroticized are widely dismissed as deficient. They are "ugly" or "sensible"—read: masculine. There is something fundamentally wrong with a woman if she prefers desexualized shoes, according to this logic, and a proper woman's shoe has sex appeal.

Third, the psychoanalytical literature shows us that women's high-heeled shoes serve multiple sexual and gender identity functions. They reassure the wearer that she is feminine yet also in possession of a kind of phallic power, which she otherwise is forced to suppress. They may too serve as a reminder of closeness with her mother. For some men, women's high-heeled shoes soothe the unconscious fear of castration and reassure that no matter how powerful women may become, they are ultimately hobbled by restrictive footwear. As Havelock Ellis wrote in the 1930s in his psychological study on sexuality, the appearance of a woman being physically restricted by her shoes—either through an explicit bondage reference, such as ankle straps, or through an implicit reference, such as a very high heel—is erotic to many people.[81]

For both women and men, then, high-heeled shoes are fetish objects in that they allay sexual anxieties and affirm gender identity.

Thus, the wearing of high-heeled shoes reinforces stereotypical ideas of what it means to be feminine and masculine, what it means to be queer and straight, what it means to be subordinated and powerful.

For this reason, it is nearly impossible to have a rational dialogue with women about making sensible footwear choices. Women resist switching from foot-deforming high heels to foot-friendly comfort shoes because they believe that their heels have a magical power. They fetishize their shoes. It's also not in the interest of men to persuade women to make the switch because they also benefit psychically from women wearing toe-crushing shoes.

In his book *The Denial of Death,* Ernest Becker offered a different paradigm. To him, fetish objects are mechanisms that help us overcome a universal anxiety—the fear of dying. The foot in particular is a stark and constant reminder of our mortality. It is the part of the body that is closest to the ground, where we will end up after we die, and it is dirty and despised, an indication of the decay of the flesh. A woman's shoe—elegant, smooth, architectural—contrasts with the foot and thereby serves as the most effective concealment of the horrible truth of our mortality. The shoe, Becker

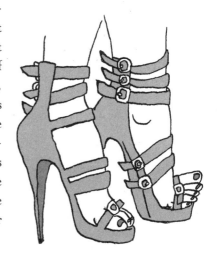

wrote, "is the closest thing *to* the body and yet is not *the* body, and it is associated with what almost always strikes fetishists as the most ugly thing: the despised foot with its calloused toes and yellowed toenails. The foot is the absolute and unmitigated testimonial to our degraded animality, to the incongruity between our proud, rich, lively, infinitely transcendent, free inner spirit and our earth-bound body. . . . Freud thought that the shoe was fetishized because, as it was the last thing the child saw before looking up at the dreaded genitals, he could safely stop there for his denial. But the foot is its own horror; what is more, it is accompanied by its own striking and transcending denial and contrast—the shoe. . . . The shoe has straps, buckles, the softest leather, the most elegant curved arch, the hardest, smoothest, shiniest heel. There is nothing like the spiked high heel in all of nature, I venture. In a word, here is the quintessence of cultural contrivance and contrast, so different from the body that it takes one a safe world away from it even while remaining intimately associated to it."[82]

Becker's theory makes particular sense today. Heels are higher than ever in the United States during a time when terrorism is a very real threat to us all. It could be that this is not a coincidence. Designers are offering fantasy shoes and women are wearing them as a way to work through anxieties. The rational thing to do, given today's political reality, is to switch to sensible shoes that enable mobility. But reason has nothing to do with women's footwear choices.

For women's shoes to be effective in keeping our anxieties—whether about sexuality or mortality—at bay, they must have a certain appearance we associate with fashionable heeled shoes. "Sensible" or sexless women's shoes don't serve any anxiety-reducing function. They do not soothe us and they do not reinforce traditional gender identities. In fact, "sensible" shoes (wide enough to wiggle your toes, stable enough to walk quickly or run in) do exactly the opposite: they subvert traditional categories of masculine and feminine. The word for lesbian in Brazil is *sapatão,* which means "big shoe." Since many heterosexual women do not want to be confused for lesbians, they refuse to wear big or sensible shoes. Lesbians who also choose to look stereotypically feminine likewise spurn "big shoes."

In his book *The Sex Life of the Foot and Shoe,* William A. Rossi explored every sexual meaning you could think of—and a lot more that you wouldn't think about—in connection with women's footwear. Rossi, a Massachusetts podiatrist and historian, died in 2003, but his book lives on as the "bible" of men's shoe fetishism.[83] It appears that Rossi loved women's footwear but did not think very highly about women as human beings. According to Rossi, women who wear "sexless" shoes are mostly "sexually turned-off women: the elderly or infirm; women of certain religious callings or members of service organizations such as Salvation Army lassies, Mennonites and Amish, etc.; or women with serious foot ills. Then there are those women with psychosexual inhibitions or neurotic problems, who use their desexed shoes as a pedic chastity belt. Or butch-type lesbians who deliberately masculinize their appearance."[84]

Rossi goes on to name Eleanor Roosevelt as a singular example of a member of this group because she believed that "sensible shoes make comfort sense." He met with Roosevelt's shoemaker, who held up for Rossi a custom-made pair of Roosevelt's shoes. Rossi took one look at the "drab, low-heeled oxfords" and "said wryly, 'You can't tell whether these are for Franklin or Eleanor.'"[85] To Rossi, any woman who chooses not to sexualize her appearance—even (or perhaps especially) a woman who is a great leader—is repressed and abnormal.

Rossi, as you have probably figured out by now, wanted all women to walk around in high-heeled shoes. He believed that women's shoes should have a "skin-tight" fit with a "pointed or tapered toe" which is "an undisputed phallic symbol." He was partial to "seminakedness" in women's feet and therefore celebrated the mule, which leaves "the foot half dressed and half undressed" with a "half-open, half-closed look" that is "designed on the same principle as the see-through blouse or dress." He also had a particular preference for "d'Orsay pumps with low-cut sides" and shoes with "deep-cut throatlines that expose toe cleavage"—again, because this look is "half-dressed, half-undressed." But the most important element is the high heel. "The higher, slimmer, and more contoured the heel, the sexier," he wrote. "This makes the foot look smaller, the arch and instep curvier, the leg longer and shapelier, the hips and buttocks wigglier. Such heels sensualize the body lines and gait."[86] Rossi also noted that, as the sex researcher Alfred Kinsey had observed, the high heel is a reminder that women arch their feet when they are sexually aroused.[87]

Notice that the foot appearing small is the first item Rossi mentions as desirable. Women are willing to endure the pain of fashionable shoes not only because they fetishize these shoes but also because they seek to fool the eyes of others in an attempt to make their feet appear tiny. A tiny shoe that encases what presumably is a tiny foot heightens the sexual fetish.

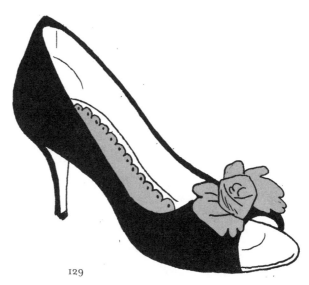

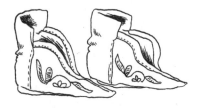

The Girl with the Tiny Feet Wins the Prince

THE ALLURE of a woman's diminutive feet has long been established. It is the centerpiece of "Cinderella," the most well-known folktale ever recorded. There are hundreds of variants of the tale; the most ancient version is from ninth-century China. Elements change but there is one constant in every version: the shoe test. In the version published by the German linguists and folklorists Jacob Grimm and Wilhelm Grimm in 1812, the protagonist is named Aschenputtel ("Ash Girl"), and the tiny, dainty shoe that slips off her foot as she flees the prince and the ball is made of solid gold. The next morning, the prince comes to her home and tells her father, "Nobody else shall be my wife but the girl whose foot this shoe fits."

The two stepsisters are thrilled because they assume they will fit into it. The eldest goes to her room with the shoe but can't fit her big toe in, because the shoe is too small for her. Her mother, Ash Girl's stepmother, hands the eldest stepsister a knife and says, "Cut the toe off; once you're queen, you won't have to walk anymore." So the stepsister cuts off her big toe, forces her foot into the shoe, and in a great deal of pain, goes out to the king's son, who assumes that she is his rightful bride. He takes her on his horse. But on the way to the castle, they pass by the grave of Ash Girl's mother, and two pigeons that had been watching over Ash Girl and had been sitting on a nearby hazel bush cry out,

"Look, look!

There's blood in the shoe!

The shoe's too small.

The right bride's still at home."

The prince looks at the stepsister's foot and sees the blood oozing out. He turns the horse around and returns to her home since she obviously is not the correct bride. Then the other sister tries on the gold shoe. She goes into her room and gets her toes in, but her heel does not fit. Her mother hands her a knife and says, "Cut a piece off your heel; once you're queen you won't have to walk anymore." The girl cuts a piece off her heel, forces her foot into the shoe, and in a great deal of pain, goes out to the king's son, who assumes that she is his rightful bride. He takes her on his horse. As they pass the hazel bush the pigeons cry out,

"Look, look!
There's blood in the shoe!
The shoe's too small.
The right bride's still at home."

He looks down at her foot and sees the blood oozing out, which is dyeing her white stockings red.

The prince takes this sister back to her home and asks the father and stepmother if there is another daughter. They admit there is Ash Girl, but say it is impossible for her to be the bride (since they had no idea she had attended the ball at which the shoe slipped off, and besides, she had no fine clothes or shoes). But the prince insists on seeing her. After Ash Girl washes her face and hands and curtsies the prince, he hands her the gold shoe. It fits her perfectly. He looks into her face and recognizes her as the girl he'd danced with and says, "That's the right bride!" He takes Ash Girl on his horse and rides off with her. When they pass the hazel bush, the pigeons cry out,

"Look, look!
No blood in the shoe!

> The shoe's not too small.
> He's bringing the right bride home."[88]

MUCH HAS been made about the fact that in the sanitized, bloodless version of the folktale recorded by the French author Charles Perrault in 1696, which is the most popular of all the variants, the slipper is glass. There has been a disagreement among folklorists over whether Perrault made an error when using the word *"verre"* (glass) when he should have used *"vair"* (fur) and that the slippers in the classic French version were truly made of fur. However, there are other non-French versions that also refer to glass slippers.[89] From our point of view—looking at Cinderella's slipper as a symbol of her genitals—glass makes perfect sense. Glass is a common symbol of virginity, since it is fragile and can be broken only one time. It would make sense for the virginal Cinderella to have tiny feet encased in glass slippers for this would reinforce the sexual fetish symbolism that underpins the tale. The perfect fit of the glass slipper represents the perfect sexual fit between the virginal Cinderella and her prince.

It is well known that Chinese women historically initiated a ritual of deliberately molding the foot to make it tiny—that is to say, they artificially created tiny feet to fit the feminine ideal in a practice not that dissimilar to the desperate antics of Cinderella's stepsisters. This practice is known as footbinding. It is a cliché in the West to claim that Chinese footbinding was horribly oppressive to women and, moreover, evidence of a kinky sexual fetish. In 1927, Freud wrote about "the Chinese custom of mutilating the female foot and then revering it like a fetish after it has been mutilated. It seems as though the Chinese male wants to thank the woman for having submitted to being castrated."[90]

The commonly held Western account of Chinese footbinding goes like this: It took place from the tenth century through the twentieth. It involved a painful and ongoing procedure that began when a girl was between five and seven years old. Her four small toes were pushed down beneath the ball of her foot, leaving only the big toe to protrude. The bones of the four small toes were broken. The forefoot and the heel were pushed together and bound tightly with wrappings. Over a period of several years, tight bandages were wound around her feet, pulling the ball and heel of the foot close together. New and tighter bindings were applied each day. The arch of the foot became clefted. By the time she was an adolescent, the foot was completely and irrevocably misshapen, and measured only a few inches in length (ideally not more than three inches from toe to heel), but she continued to tightly bind her feet to maintain the size and shape for the rest of her life. Chinese women created vibrantly colored, embroidered silk slippers that, together with the bindings, concealed the foot and added to its mystery.

The foot itself was said to resemble a "golden lotus" plant and was held up as an erotic and feminine ideal. It is said that Chinese men revered the "lotus foot," whose big toe resembled a phallus and whose cleft in the sole resembled a vagina, and that women with bound feet walked (by necessity) in mincing steps. Their gait was considered sexy and alluring.

Girls submitted to this painful and debilitating procedure because it marked them as ideal wives and they worried that if they remained unbound they would never marry. Many girls suffered from infections, which sometimes led to their deaths and always led to lifelong pains. Older women were susceptible to falls, leading to fractures of the hip and other bones.

Footbinding was outlawed in 1912 but continued for several decades afterward. It is estimated that between 50 million and 4.5 billion women had their feet bound.[91]

Over the past decade, fascinating scholarship has complicated this narrative. The overall outline is not inaccurate, and the oppression and sexual meanings are undeniable. But the Western account does not tell the whole story. Dorothy Ko, a professor of history at Barnard, has been frustrated that a heterogeneous, multilayered practice, spanning a millennium and many different provinces, has been reduced to the lowest common denominators that reinforce racist stereotypes about Asian women as submissive and eroticized. In fact, she wrote, "footbinding was not a uniform practice—both the technique of binding and its meaning changed with time and place. Although there is not one cause for footbinding but many, it remained the single most important experience in a woman's life between the thirteenth and nineteenth centuries."[92]

Freud viewed footbinding from a male perspective of castration anxiety. Ko, however, situates it from the perspective of the mothers who enforced it and the daughters who submitted to it. An elaborate set of rituals around crafting shoes sprung up, and women busied themselves creating beautifully decorated slippers that showed off their artistic talents. For women, the practice created a valued identity as modest, domestic, skilled at textile work, and able to endure the pain of childbirth. Footbinding created "a bittersweet awareness that as women, they could gain power only by way of their bodies. . . . This message would soon be inscribed on the daughter's very body. . . . For a woman, the body was her only gateway to a better future. To do textile work and to give birth—to attain value and meaning for herself, she could not do without the body."[93]

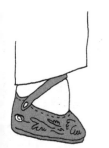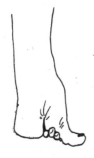

There is little historical evidence about how the practice began, but Ko maintains that it developed in the tenth century among professional dancers and then spread to the elite, upper-class Han Chinese (the majority ethnic group). It was not intended to cripple but to enhance one's grace. However, as the practice spread its meanings shifted, and by the seventeenth century even rural women were involved in it.

Western women and men often condemn footbinding as barbaric. By implication, the women who practiced it were victimized, ignorant, or self-hating. Please allow me to point out just a few of many parallels we can draw between Chinese footbinding and Western women wearing high heels:

- In both cases, the foot is permanently deformed.
- In both cases, the foot takes on an ambisexuality. The bound foot is both phallic (because only the big toe protrudes) and vagina-like (because of the deep cleft that is formed in the sole). The foot in pointy-toed high heels is also phallic (in the toe and in the heel) yet symbolic of the female genitals (because of the shoe's slender, tight shape and opening).
- In both cases, a sexual fetish object is created.
- In both cases, the practice is an assertion of femininity for the wearer and an affirmation of masculinity for the men who appreciate the practice. Heterosexuality as the norm is affirmed in both.
- In both cases, mobility is limited and the restrictive state is regarded as sexually alluring.

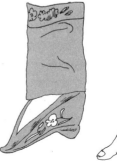
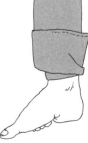

- In both cases, it is believed that a woman's value is written on her body.
- In both cases, if a woman refuses to participate in the practice, she is regarded as deficient or deviant.
- In both cases, the practice proves that one is able to handle pain and exert a sense of control and discipline over her body, demonstrating a perverse kind of strength.
- In both cases, the shoe is an instrument of illusion. Ko points out that while lotus shoes were tiny, the feet that wore them were invariably bigger and very seldom a mere three inches. Depending on the style of the shoe, the heel of the foot often did not fit into the shoe but remained outside of it. The bulk of the foot was concealed by long pants or leggings so that only the pointed toe stuck out.[94] Women wearing high heels also display their feet to look as tiny as possible: the higher the heel, the smaller the foot inside it appears because the high arch tricks the eye. Also, women jam big feet into too-small shoes and often wear long pants that conceal most of the shoe.
- In both cases, beautiful shoes disguise the horrible reality of disfigured feet. Susie Lan Cassel of California State University–San Marcos has written that the entire enterprise of creating gorgeous, embroidered, silk lotus shoes was "to keep the putrescence of the flesh a secret while calling attention to the enticingly small size of the feet. . . . The bindings . . . functioned to hide a mys-

tery too horrible to reveal," which was the "rotting foot."[95] One woman, whose mother had bound feet, told National Public Radio reporter Louisa Lim that "the bandages that women used for footbinding were about ten feet long, so it was difficult for them to wash their feet. They only washed once every two weeks, so it was very, very stinky."[96] Likewise, as high-heel-wearing women's feet become increasingly misshapen, they tend to become embarrassed to reveal their naked feet and conceal them in shoes that cause further disfigurement.

It doesn't matter whether or not you accept the psychoanalytical theory that a high heel is a sexual fetish object. What does matter is that women are deliberately shaping a part of their body into an unnatural form in order to sexualize it. When women in another time and place have done the same thing, we have denounced the practice. It is time to look at ourselves in the mirror.

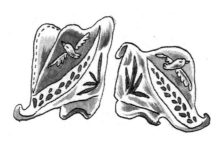

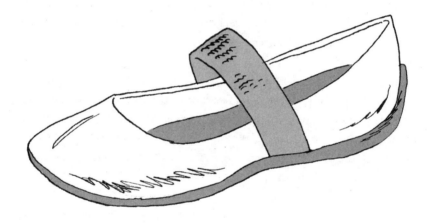

Chapter 7

SHOES WISELY
How to Shoe Shop

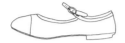

MANY ELEGANT women wear low-heeled or flat shoes to great effect. In addition to the famous fashion icons Katharine and Audrey Hepburn and Jacqueline Kennedy Onassis, chic women today such as Michelle Obama, Carla Bruni-Sarkozy, Kate Winslet, Reese Witherspoon, Sienna Miller, and Sofia Coppola routinely wear shoes with low or no heels. Even Anna Wintour, the editor in chief of *Vogue*, known for her stilettos as much as for her bobbed hair and sunglasses, has been spotted in flats.

If you're a smart shoe shopper, you can find many pairs that are fashionable, fetching, finely made, and—hold your breath—sensible. "The holy grail is a shoe with a lot of eye appeal and is comfortable, and it's getting easier and easier to find this type of shoe," says Julian Kershaw, owner of The Walk Shop in Berkeley, the first walking footwear specialty store in the US. "A lot of manufacturers today are providing both style and comfort." Here is what you need to know.

CHOOSE SHOES YOU CAN USE

- Don't buy shoes from the Internet. Go to a shoe store that specializes in old-fashioned sit-and-fit service. There are many excellent stores throughout the country that offer a wide selection of fashionable yet comfortable shoes.[97] "We always try to recommend a shoe that is both comfortable and flattering," says Brittney Rothweiler, the women's buyer for The Tannery in Boston. "Because we carry so many brands, everyone can find something."

- Since feet swell somewhat as the day goes on, shop for shoes in the afternoon.

- Ask the salesperson to measure your feet. Don't presume that you know your shoe size. As you get older, your feet become wider, longer, and stiffer. Many of us put on extra pounds as we age, which can exacerbate a number of problems because it adds even more pressure on the foot when walking.

- To make sure that you buy the right size, stand on a blank piece of paper at home and trace the outline of your feet with a pen. Bring the tracing with you when you shop for shoes; the pair you buy should cover the outline of your foot.

- Know your shoe width. It does not occur to many women that they may need a wide-sized shoe (meaning that the toe box, not the heel, is roomy). If your forefoot is significantly wider than your heel, you may need a wide size. Alternately, you may need the narrow width. Do not assume that you fit into the default medium. The good news is that many shoe manufacturers offer a number of styles in various widths. The bad news is that your local store may not stock them all. In this case, I make an exception to the "Don't use the Internet" rule. If you want to compare the medium width with a narrow or wide one, go ahead and order different widths from an online store and keep the one that fits best. Before you put your money down, make sure you can return the other pairs for a full refund.

- Even if your width is medium, make a concerted effort to shop for shoes that are wider in front, narrower in the back. If there are no such shoes in the store, leave.

- One foot is usually larger than the other. Buy shoes to match the size of the larger foot. Ask the salesperson to insert a pad, if necessary, in the shoe of the smaller foot.

- Make sure you can wiggle all your toes. This is possible if you wear shoes with a toe box that is rounded or squared, not pointed. Make sure there is at least a quarter inch between the end of your longest toe (either your big toe or your second toe) and the end of the shoe.

- "People usually only try on one shoe and they don't walk

around as much as they need to see if it fits," advises Danny Wasserman, a veteran shoe salesman and owner of Tip Top Shoes in New York City. "If the shoes can be returned, take home two pairs and walk around on your carpet to see which one fits best."

- Make sure the heel doesn't ride up and down as you walk. If it does, ask the salesperson to insert a pad to make the fit snug.
- The upper should be soft and breathable. The sole should be firm, though with some cushioning, to protect the foot from the shock of concrete and other hard surfaces. It should be slightly flexible, able to bend at the toe box, but never so flexible that it's capable of folding or twisting.
- Not everyone needs arch support. But if you overpronate—and if you are like 70 percent of the population, you do—you should wear shoes with built-in support or an orthotic or over-the-counter insert as much as possible. This is also true for people with high arches. (See page 153, on orthotics and inserts.)
- When you're in the store, walk around in the shoes on a hard, uncarpeted surface. Chances are that the store has carpeting with extra-thick padding beneath it. But once you're outside the store, you are most likely to walk on hard surfaces.
- Don't look for a bargain by choosing shoes that are cheaply made—although if you see a high-quality shoe marked down on sale that fits and looks good, of course you should grab

it! Cheaply manufactured shoes have too-thin soles, inadequate cushioning, and stiff uppers. They also lack arch support and contoured insoles. Better to have one pair of well-made shoes than two pairs that are poorly constructed.

- Don't wear the same pair or even the same style every day. If you do, you will apply repeated pressure on specific areas of your foot that may lead to pain or deformity. Rotating shoes also allows them to air out.

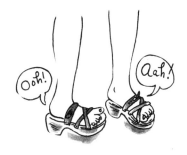

SMART SANDALS

- When the weather is warm, wear sandals when possible. They emancipate your toes from the tyranny of the closed-toe shoes you're forced to wear in cold weather.
- Make sure your feet are securely kept in place and that the straps do not cut into your skin.
- Look for styles with contoured foot beds offering some arch support.

- If you wear orthotics, choose sandals with removable insoles. Place the orthotic in the space where the insole normally sits. You might have to loosen or tighten straps to accommodate the height difference between the insole that came with the sandal and the orthotic with which you're replacing it.

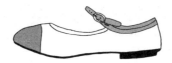

THESE SHOES WERE MADE FOR SERIOUS WALKING
- For everyday walking, choose a shoe with a heel between a half inch to an inch.
- Lace-up or Velcro styles are best for everyday walking because you can tighten or loosen them to get a custom fit.
- If you wear sneakers or athletic shoes on a regular basis, you will cut your risk of foot pain later in life by more than half (when compared with women who wear regular shoes).[98]

THE LOW DOWN ON HIGH HEELS
- Don't believe the shoe hype that you have to go higher than three and a half inches to have a "high" heel. Keep heel heights in perspective: A heel that is one inch or lower is low heeled. A heel that is between one to two inches is mid-height. A heel

that is two inches and higher classifies as high. A heel that is four inches or higher is demented. You don't need to go higher than two inches to achieve a flattering, leggy look.

- Save high-heeled shoes, which force the feet into unnatural positions, for special occasions, and don't walk far in them. "Try to limit the amount of time you wear high heels to three hours at a time," advises Dr. Carol Frey. "Kick them off when possible. Try to find shoes that are not over two and a half inches at the heel. They should have buttery-soft leather uppers or woven patterns that have some 'give' as the skin gets warmer."

- The higher the heel, the more pressure is placed on the forefoot, the higher the likelihood of developing a bunion, bunionette, hammertoe, neuroma, corn, or callus. According to one study, a three-quarter-inch heel increases forefoot plantar (underside of the foot) pressure by 22 percent (when compared with no heel). But a two-inch heel increases the pressure by 57 percent. And a three-and-a-quarter-inch heel increases the pressure by 76 percent.[99] Another study found that the change from a sneaker to a three-inch-heeled shoe increases forefoot pressure to 110 percent.[100] No matter how you crunch the numbers, your toes are indisputably being crunched.

- If your profession requires you to wear heels, limit the height to as low as you can get away with.

- When possible, opt for a rounded toe. Open-toe or peep-toe styles tend to be most comfortable with high heels.
- Avoid a pointed forefoot that squeezes your toes. If you must have the pointy look, make sure your toes lie within the widest part of the toe box and that your foot is not forced too far forward into the shoe.
- Make sure the front of your foot doesn't slide forward when you walk. There should be cushioning beneath the ball of the foot, because that is the place where you apply the most pressure when you wear high heels.
- Choose a thick heel, not a stiletto, for stability.
- If you must wear heels during the day, bring a backup pair in a lower height and alternate your shoes whenever possible. If you wear high heels every day without a break, you run the risk of shortening your Achilles tendons.

THE BAD SHOE HALL OF FAME

- Beware of stiletto mules: your foot could fall out or you could twist your ankle. If you must have this look, find a pair with a strap across the midfoot to secure your foot.
- Platforms should be low or mid-height. It's easy to lose your balance while wearing high platforms, leading to a twisted ankle. High platform sandals in particular can be treacherous because there is no heel counter to grip and stabilize your heel.

- Don't purchase ballet slippers unless they have a contoured foot bed or built-in arch support or you can insert your own orthotics. Soles that are completely flat can cause feet to roll inward. If you covet the pancake-flat look, consider a pair with a strap across the midfoot, such as a Mary Jane style, to hold your foot in place. If you wear long pants, no one will see the strap.

- Save flip-flops and slides for the beach or pool, and don't walk in them for long distances. They can cause tendonitis and plantar fasciitis. "You really shouldn't wear flip-flops when you're walking around unless you just had a pedicure and you're walking home," says Dr. Johanna Youner. "Flip-flops have single-handedly caused more problems with people's feet in the last couple years than probably any other type of shoe," warns Dr. Rock Positano. The problem with flip-flops and slides is that "the foot is able to go in any direction it wants to go in, and it directly impairs the ability of the foot to function as a shock-absorbing part of the body."[101]

- Be wary of any sandal or shoe that promises to contribute to weight loss by toning the calf, thigh, and gluteal muscles. A very popular brand of flip-flops claims to be "footwear with a gym built in" and that you can "get a workout while you walk." This is marketing, not medicine, speaking. All flip-flops, even those with thick soles and contoured foot beds, fail to hold the foot in place and therefore should not be worn for more than very short periods of time.

• "Rocker sole" shoes are not for everyone. They are claimed to work the wearer's gluteal muscles, to correct her posture, and to alleviate foot, knee, and back problems. This type of shoe is heavy and oversized, with a rocker bottom that causes the feet to roll through each step. "They're very good for a certain patient population," says Dr. Youner. "But I think it's a fallacy that they give you an extra level of fitness. They're good for stretching out the back of your legs. But you can get tendonitis if you're not careful. You should ask your podiatrist and let her decide." The same is true of "negative heel" shoes, in which the heel sits lower than the toes.

• At home, don't wear flimsy slippers. Instead, wear shoes with a contoured foot bed and/or arch support. It doesn't matter if you think this type of shoe is hideously ugly. When you're alone or with family, who cares what your shoes look like anyway? If you have no major foot problems, clogs or other slip-on, backless styles (that have the ease of slippers) with built-in support are good choices.

• Sheepskin-lined boots and moccasins are comfortable and cozy—at first. But their soles are too flexible, making the foot and ankle work too hard to walk. Either insert arch support (see page 153) or save them for lounging when you're not walking anywhere and you just want to keep your feet toasty.

CUSTOMIZE YOUR SHOES

• If you have a pair of heels you adore that you refuse to relinquish despite the pain, modify them. For those who can afford the $250 price tag, the "shoe surgery" performed at Eneslow, the Foot Comfort Center, in New York City, is almost as good as getting a custom-made pair of shoes. The technicians at Eneslow take your existing pair and redesign it to provide more toe room, reduce the slope of the heel, and relieve pressure to the ball of your foot, among other changes. Suze Yalof Schwartz, the executive fashion editor of *Glamour* magazine, brought a pair of sparkly gold Manolo Blahnik stilettos to Eneslow for a complete overhaul. They were widened an inch, given memory foam insoles, had the heel cut down by a quarter of an inch, and were given a thicker sole. According to Schwartz, the visual changes were so subtle that no one could tell the difference, but now her favorite shoes, which she never used to wear because they pinched her feet after wearing them for ten minutes, feel "amazing." To watch the transformation, go to http://www.glamour.com/fashion/blogs/slaves-to-fashion/2009/08/shoe-makeovers-say-au-revoir-t.html.[102] You can see for yourself that even shoe surgery did not eliminate Schwartz's toe cleavage.

- Your local shoe repairman may also be able to stretch the toe box to accommodate a wide forefoot, shave off a half inch from the heel, and insert cushioning. To find someone good, call or visit a high-end shoe boutique and ask the manager where the store sends its merchandise in need of repair.

- There are affordable options too. Visit a shoe repair shop, drugstore, or athletics store and you will discover an array of inexpensive over-the-counter shoe inserts. If the ball of your foot hurts, try a metatarsal cushion made of gel, foam, or moleskin. For high heels or sandals, try the extra-thin adhesive cushions from Solemate (*www.highheelshurt.com*). If your heel is giving you trouble, experiment with a heel cushion. If the heel of the shoe is too wide and you step out of the shoe, try heel liners. There are bunion cushions and callus cushions too. You have to be willing to experiment to see what works best, but as a general rule, the shoe you are customizing must not be too tight or there won't be any space for the inserts. You can also buy over-the-counter insoles. Bring these with you when you go shoe shopping and try them on together with the shoes you are considering for purchase.

SKIRT SHOES VS. PANT SHOES

- When you're wearing pants, wear low-heeled shoes. You can hide most of the shoe if you hem your pants long. Ergo, unless you are attending a special or dressy event, don't wear high-heeled shoes with pants. There just isn't enough beauty benefit to this look that would justify the potential deformation you are causing your feet.

- Save your narrower, higher-heeled shoes to wear with skirts. A wide, chunky shoe looks fine with a full or A-line skirt, but a daintier shoe with some height best completes an outfit with a pencil skirt. Look for shoes with a kitten heel (a thin heel of one and a half to two inches) and a rounded toe or a moderate platform or wedge for everyday wear.

ORTHOTICS VS. OVER-THE-COUNTER INSERTS

BEFORE THE Industrial Revolution, when shoes were made by hand, shoemakers constructed shoes around the actual foot of the wearer. Therefore, shoes were made with built-in arch support when it was needed. But now that shoes are mass made, it is up to us to tailor our shoes ourselves using products that slip inside our shoes.

An orthotic (sometimes called an orthosis) is a custom-made shoe insert. Your doctor measures your foot in just a few minutes by either taking a cast mold of your foot or taking a digital image of your arch and heel pattern. A lab manufactures the insert and your doctor gives it to you with instructions on how often to wear it. The orthotic is made of a firm material with a cushioned cover. You put the orthotic

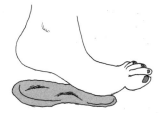

inside your shoe with your foot on top of it. In the beginning you may be aware of the sensation of having something extra in your shoe, but that feeling goes away quickly.

Not everyone needs an orthotic. They are prescribed primarily for those with bunions associated with overpronation or for those with a thin fat pad on the sole.

Your shoe should have a heel of two inches or fewer for the orthotic to work properly; ideally the heel should be closer to one inch.

The good news: orthotics last for several years. The bad news: they are expensive. They cost several hundred dollars each, and many insurance companies do not cover the cost even when medically indicated.

An over-the-counter insert is a prefabricated, non-customized orthotic. It is sold in sporting goods stores and online. Dr. Johanna Youner recommends the Superfeet, Spenco, and Powerstep brands. "Posture control" inserts from Posture Dynamics can be ordered online (*www.mortonsfoot.com*), and Dr. Scholl's also makes well-made insoles that are sold in chain drugstores. Sometimes inserts are referred to as "foot beds," "arch supports," or "insoles." They are significantly cheaper than orthotics—typically costing between $30 to $50—but they only last a few months and then need to be replaced.

The several-hundred-dollar question: Do you need customized orthotics, or can you get away with over-the-counter inserts? According to Dr. Carol Frey, "It's okay to start with an over-the-counter product. There are some good ones that are available and they're worth trying." For most people, adds Youner, "You don't need custom unless you have real problems or you're a runner. They are too expensive and they don't really work for high heels anyway."

A new, three-year study, announced in June 2009 and sponsored by the American Podiatric Medical Association, is investigating the success rate of orthotics in treating heel pain and is comparing customized orthotics with over-the-counter inserts. It is the first study of its kind to measure how specific foot types—such as those with high and low arches—respond to orthotics and inserts.[103]

I overpronate and have bunions. My goal is to slow down or even halt the development of my bunions by altering the biomechanics of my gait. I've chosen orthotics instead of the over-the-counter option. They cost much more but they also last significantly longer, so in the end the price difference is not big, although the up-front price differential is tremendous.

I wear my orthotics all the time at home. Instead of slippers, I wear backless leather sandals with thick straps across the midfoot that adjust with Velcro. The shoes came with removable foot beds so I went ahead and removed them. My orthotics start at the heel but end before the toes, so I took a pair of inexpensive, flat, drugstore insoles, cut out the forefoot area, and placed them in the sandals so that my toes have a soft surface on which to rest.

Outside of my home, I try to wear orthotics at least half the time. This isn't always easy, since shoes that accommodate orthotics tend to have a sporty look and that isn't always the style I'm going for, particularly when I wear a skirt or dress. When I don't wear orthotics, I usually wear shoes with built-in arch support. I save my high-heeled (two and a half inches at most) non-orthotic, unsupported shoes for dressed-up occasions just a few hours two times a week, three times at most.

Whichever option you choose, you need to know a few facts:

- Different types of shoes require different-sized orthotics or inserts. Sneakers need wide orthotics/inserts while dress shoes need narrow ones. I own three pairs of orthotics: for sneakers/wide walking shoes; for narrow, heeled boots (with the heels not higher than two inches); and for shoes that are medium in width. I brought several pairs of shoes and boots to my podiatrist when he measured my feet, and he sent them to the lab along with my casts. (Yes, I got them back.)

- Orthotics/inserts work best in shoes with removable insoles. Otherwise, they create too much height inside your shoe and your foot will step out of it when you walk. If your orthotic/insert is not full length (for example, if it ends before your toes), you should cut the removable insole to leave only the toe area inside the shoe. (If you don't want to do this yourself, find a good shoe repair person and ask him to do it for you.) That way you will have cushioning for the part of your foot not covering the orthotic/insert.

- You place the orthotic in your shoe by aligning it against the inside of the heel. Thus, you need a shoe with a back. The only way to wear orthotics/inserts with backless shoes is by removing the insole. If the insole is not removable, you're out of luck. Even if you can fit the orthotic/insole into the shoe, you might find your foot stepping out of the shoe if there is no strap holding your foot in place.

- The tighter the shoe, the less likely there will be room for an orthotic/insert. You might have to go up a half size or just save tighter shoes for special occasions when you forego the orthotic/insert.

- Pumps and ballet slippers without a strap across the foot generally can't accommodate orthotics/inserts. Lace-up shoes, Mary Jane—style shoes with a strap across the midstep, boots, and even sandals with straps (preferably adjustable) are better because they prevent your foot from stepping out of the shoe.

- You have to experiment and take your time buying new shoes to gauge whether or not they will work for you. Bring your orthotics/inserts with you to the store and try them on with the shoes. This new way of shoe shopping is a plus: you won't be tempted to make an impulse purchase you'll regret later.

RECOMMENDED MANUFACTURERS

IT IS increasingly common to find "good for you" shoes with a touch of "bad shoe" style. Look for these labels, and note that many of them manufacture shoes in various widths, from narrow to extra-wide:

AEROSOLES	DONALD PLINER	PRADA
ANYI LU	EASY SPIRIT	RIEKER
ARA	ECCO	ROCKPORT
ARCHE	FINN COMFORT	SALVATORE FERRAGAMO
ARCOPEDICO	HELLE COMFORT	SANITA
BEAUTIFEEL	KEEN	SÖFFT
BIRKENSTOCK	MEPHISTO	STUART WEITZMAN
BRUNO MAGLI	MERRELL	TARYN ROSE
BORN	MUNRO	THIERRY RABOTIN
LA CANADIENNE	NATURALIZER	THINK!
CLARKS	NAOT	WOLKY[104]
COLE HAAN	OH! SHOES	
DANSKO	PAUL GREEN	

Why Do Big-Name Designer Shoes Cost So Much?

I ASKED several people to explain the enormous price difference between expensive designer shoes, such as those from Stuart Weitzman (typically $250 to $300), versus stratospherically expensive shoes made by the likes of Jimmy Choo, Manolo Blahnik, and Christian Louboutin ($600 to $1200). Does the extra money buy a better shoe?

Dr. Johanna Youner:
"The materials are finer with Jimmy Choos and Manolos, but they are definitely not more comfortable than Stuart Weitzmans. I was given a pair of four-inch Manolo Blahniks as a gift years ago. I wore them recently for a professional appearance. After an hour I took them off and put them in my bag. No way are they comfortable. They are very elegant. My feet looked gorgeous. But after an hour I was dying.

"Some of the Stuart Weitzman lines are very functional with high and wide toe boxes. They are very good for every day. They cost a few hundred dollars, but you need to spend that kind of money to get a comfortable high heel."

Forty-four-year-old designer-shoe wearer:

"My feet feel more secure in the high-end designer shoes, even when they're strappy. They just feel cradled better. But maybe it's because I think they're cradled better. When I walk in them for a few hours, my feet start to hurt so much I feel like I can't take another step. Maybe there's not such a big difference between the $300 shoes and the $900 shoes. It could be that when you have these fabulous shoes, you walk with an extra bounce in your step."

Twenty-six-year-old shoe lover:

"I could never justify to myself getting a pair of designer shoes because of the price. I eyed this one pair of gold flats, and my mother bought it for me as a present. I was so excited. I wore them three times and I was in agony. My feet felt like they were burning—on the sides and in the toes. I was surprised because I figured they were high quality."

Elizabeth Semmelhack, author of *Heights of Fashion* and chief curator of the Bata Shoe Museum in Toronto:

"When you buy $1,200 Stella McCartneys you are getting $1,200 worth of social status. The value you're getting is

> **not that the shoes are comfortable or long lasting. What you're getting is $1,200 worth of momentary social standing. It's momentary because next season you have to buy the next pair."**

IN RECOMMENDING that you reconsider your footwear choices, I am most certainly not suggesting that you "let yourself go" in the name of comfort, or that it doesn't really matter what shoes you wear because "it's inner beauty that counts." Not at all. It is my belief that making an effort to look pleasing demonstrates respect for oneself and for others.

All I am saying is that when choosing shoes to wear during the day, don't hold a too-narrow idea of what "pretty" or "sexy" or "flattering" is. Take a fresh look. Reevaluate and expand your perspective.

You want to wear your fancy, fantastical, fetishistic shoes? No problem—but save them for special occasions. Wear them sparingly and judiciously.

"There is a lot of emotion when you're intending to buy a pair of shoes you love, and you can lose control," says Robert Schwartz, president and CEO of Eneslow. "But you can get to a certain point in life when you realize that what's most important is how you feel physically, not just emotionally, including how to improve your posture and your alignment. When you get to that point, you are empowered, and you realize that your sexuality is less about getting men to notice your shoes and more about what your eyes express. Then you will feel great and have enhanced your own self-esteem."

When a woman is crisp and well groomed, and walks with a jaunty, confident gait, she is a force to be reckoned with. She is unequivocally not sexy when she hobbles in shoes that mold her toes into overlapping claws. Yes, it's true that gorgeous shoes can transform an outfit from simple to sensational, but you can just as easily add visual interest with a colorful scarf, a chunky necklace, bold earrings, a waist-nipping belt . . . or (best of all) a smile that tells the world that you take care of yourself and that *you* know you look enchanting.

If you put head over heels, your feet will remain in excellent shape and take you wherever you want to go. What could be more alluring than that?

Notes

1   Amy Odell, "Two Models Fall, Many Stumble at Prada," September 24, 2008, reported in *New York* magazine and other news outlets, available online at *http://nymag.com/daily/fashion/2008/09/two_models_fall_many_more_stum.html*.

2   StyleCaster, "Brian Reyes Fall 2009: Not So Well-Heeled," February 19, 2009, available online at *http://www.stylecaster.com/rss/152533/brian-reyes-fall-2009-not-so-well-heeled*.

3   Lisa Armstrong, "Head Over Heels: Bigger Is Better For This Season's Crop of Over-The-Top Stilettos and Other Teetering Treasures," *Harper's Bazaar*, March 2009, 241.

4   André Leon Talley, "Keep It Short," *Vogue.com*, June 10, 2009, available online at *http://www.style.com/vogue/voguedaily/2009/06/keep-it-short/*.

5   The survey was conducted by Kelton Research for the American Podiatric Medical Association and involved 500 women. Cited in Catherine Saint Louis, "The Secret Is Out: We Can See Your Feet," *New York Times*, August 6, 2009, E1.

6   *APMA Foot Ailments Survey*, January 2009. The results are available online at *www.apma.org*.

7   Michael J. Coughlin, "Women's Shoe Wear and Foot Disorders," *Western Journal of Medicine* (December 1995) 163.6:569–570.

8   Tribble Ad Agency, "Flip Flops," November 5, 2007, available online at *http://www.tribbleagency.com?p=442*.

9   Glenn Copeland, DPM, Stan Solomon, and Mark Myerson, MD, *The Good Foot Book: A Guide For Men, Women, Children, Athletes, Seniors—Everyone* (Alameda, CA: Hunter, 2005), 185.

10   *AOFAS Position Statement*, "Cosmetic Foot Surgery," available online at *www.aofas.org*.

11   *APMA High Heels Survey*, 2003. A national sample of 503 women ages eighteen and older was surveyed by telephone to collect the data. The findings are available online at *www.apma.org*.

12   *AOFAS Position Statement*, "Women's Shoes and Foot Problems," available online at *www.aofas.org*.

13   The wife of Ferdinand Marcos, the Philippine dictator, Imelda Marcos never had to worry about matching the right shoes to her outfit. In 1986, when the Marcos regime was toppled, it was discovered that she possessed 2,700 pairs of designer shoes.

14   In a different context, empty shoes are symbols of horror. Photographs of mountains of shoes, taken from Jews and other minorities who were gassed and then burned by the Nazis during the Holocaust, are potent because we can easily visualize the people who owned the shoes. It is obvious that those shoes were worn by actual women, men, and children, whom we know were systematically murdered. A photograph of a pile of the victims' pants or shirts would also elicit horror, but not quite as powerfully. This is because pants and shirts lose their shape after they are removed from the body; they do not evoke the same bodily sense of the wearer. For further exploration, see Jeffrey Feldman's excellent essay "The Holocaust Shoe: Untying Memory: Shoes as Holocaust Memorial Experience" in *Jews and Shoes*, ed. Edna Nahshon (Oxford and New York: Berg, 2008), 119–130. Empty shoes also have been used strategically as a political statement to evoke a sense of horror at the loss of human life. In 1994 in Washington, D.C., forty

thousand pairs of shoes were arrayed around the Capitol Reflecting Pool in symbolic testimony to people killed each year by gunshots in murders, suicides, and accidents. In France, thousands of empty shoes have been piled into pyramids to raise awareness of the hundreds of thousands of civilians killed by land mines.

15   Quoted by Courtney Rubin, "Sarah Jessica Parker Has Stiletto Woes," August 2, 2007, available online at *http://www.people.com/people/article/0,,20049430,00.html*.

16   *Shoeblog.com*, "I've Got A Bone To Pick With You, SJP," March 12, 209, available online at *http://www.shoeblog.com/blog/ive-got-a-bone-to-pick-with-you-sjp/*.

17   New York Radical Women, "No More Miss America," in *Dear Sisters: Dispatches From the Women's Liberation Movement*, eds. Rosalyn Baxandall and Linda Gordon (New York: Basic, 2000), 184.

18   Marcelle Karp and Debbie Stoller, eds., *The Bust Guide to the New Girl Order* (New York: Penguin, 1999), 3, 6.

19   Karp and Stoller, 43, 47.

20   For example, see Tace Hedrick, "Are You a *Pura Latina*? Or, Menudo Every Day: *Tacones* and Symbolic Ethnicity," in *Footnotes: On Shoes*, eds. Shari Benstock and Suzanne Ferriss (New Brunswick, NJ and London: Rutgers University), 135–155.

21   Sandra Bernhard and Annie Leibovitz, "Why High Heels?" *New Yorker*, February 26, 1996, 192, available online at http://www.newyorker.com.

22   "Feet Hurt? Stop Wearing Shoes," National Public Radio, April 22, 2008, transcript available online at *www.npr.org*.

23   Carol Frey, "Foot Health and Shoewear for Women," *Clinical Orthopaedics and Related Research* vol. 372 (March 2000): 32–44.

24   Copeland and Solomon, 17–18.

25   D. Casey Kerrigan, Mary K. Todd, and Patrick O. Riley, "Knee Osteoarthritis
      and High-Heeled Shoes," *Lancet* (May 9, 1998) 351:1399–1401; D. Casey Kerri-
      gan, Jennifer L. Johansson, Mary G. Bryant, et al., "Moderate-Heeled Shoes and
      Knee Joint Torques Relevant to the Development and Progression of Knee
      Osteoarthritis," *Archives of Physical Medicine and Rehabilitation* (May 2005): 86.5: 871–875.

26   Carol Frey, Francesca Thompson, Judith Smith, et al., "American Orthope-
      dic Foot and Ankle Society Women's Shoe Survey," *Foot and Ankle International*
      (1993) 14.2:78–81.

27   Natalie Angier, "Many Women Buy Foot Trouble with Fashionable High
      Heels," *New York Times*, March 7, 1991, available online at *http://www.nyt.com*.

28   Carol Frey, Francesca Thompson, and Judith Smith, "Update on Women's
      Footwear," *Foot and Ankle International* (1995) 16.6:328–331.

29   Hylton B. Menz and Meg E. Morris, "Footwear Characteristics and Foot
      Problems in Older People," *Gerontology* (2005) 51:346–351.

30   Printed with the permission of Carol Frey, MD, Manhattan Beach, CA.

31   Gardiner Harris, "If Shoe Won't Fit, Fix the Foot? Popular Surgery Raises
      Concern," *New York Times*, December 7, 2003, available online at *www.nytimes.com*.
      This trend had been covered several months previously in Sarah Baxter, "Fash-
      ion Victims Have Their Toes Trimmed to Fit Shoes," *Sunday Times* (London),
      August 10, 2003, available online at *www.timesonline.co.uk*.

32   Catherine Piercy, "Happy Feet," *Vogue*, April 2008, 226.

33   Irina Aleksandr, "Time for Toetox? Park Avenue Podiatrist Tends to Tor-
      tured Soles," *New York Observer*, April 10, 2009, 14.

34   Aleksandr, 13.

35   *http://www.institutebeaute.com*, accessed on August 18, 2009.

36 *AOFAS*, "Cosmetic Foot Surgery to Beautify Feet Has Serious Risks," December 29, 2004, available on *www.aofas.org*.

37 Harris, "If Shoe Won't Fit."

38 *http://www.iafs.com*, accessed on August 18, 2009.

39 Cited in Ariel Levy, *Female Chauvinist Pigs: Women and the Rise of Raunch Culture* (New York: Free Press, 2005), 195.

40 Elizabeth Semmelhack's book offers a thorough and very readable social history of "elevated" shoes (platform and high heels) in Western Europe and the United States. I have relied on the history related in her book for this section. See Elizabeth Semmelhack, *Heights of Fashion: A History of the Elevated Shoe* (Pittsburgh: Periscope, 2008). I also recommend highly, and relied upon, Caroline Cox, *Stiletto* (New York: Harper Design, 2004); and Colin McDowell, *Shoes: Fashion and Fantasy* (London: Thames and Hudson, 1989).

41 McDowell, 27.

42 Cited in McDowell, 27.

43 Maria Giuseppe Muzzarelli, "Sumptuous Shoes: Making and Wearing in Medieval Italy," in *Shoes: A History From Sandals to Sneakers*, eds. Giorgio Riello and Peter McNeil (New York and Oxford: Berg/Oxford, 2006), 68.

44 Muzzarelli, 64.

45 William A. Rossi, *The Sex Life of the Foot and Shoe* (Ware, Hertfordshire, UK: Wordsworth, 1989), 152. This book was first published by Routledge & Kegan Paul in 1977.

46 Rossi, 220.

47 Semmelhack, 21. Published in conjunction with the Bata Shoe Museum in Toronto, Canada.

48 Semmelhack, 25.

49 Mary Wollstonecraft, *Vindication of the Rights of Woman* (New York: Penguin, 1992), 132.

50 George Sand, L'Histoire de ma vie, 203–204, cited in Nancy Rexford, "The Perils of Choice: Women's Footwear in Nineteenth-Century America," in Riello and McNeil, 144.

51 See Anthony Barthelemy, "Brogans," in Benstock and Ferriss, 179–196.

52 Marc Linder and Charles L. Saltzman, "A History of Medical Scientists on High Heels," *International Journal of Health Services* (1998) 28.2: 209.

53 "Well-Dressed Suffragists," *The New York Times*, April 21, 1912. Cited in Semmelhack, 35.

54 "Fashion Blamed: Dress Reform, Not Votes, the Need of the Hour, Says Humanity Lover," *The New York Times*, March 28, 1915. Cited in Semmelhack, 35.

55 A. Magruder, "High Heels and Low Heels: The Difference Shown in X-Ray Photographs," *Ladies' Home Journal*, January 1908, 33. Cited in Linder and Saltzman, 211–212.

56 "Lay the High Heel Low," *The Washington Post*, May 6, 1920. Cited in Semmelhack, 40.

57 Cited in Maureen Reilly, *Hot Shoes: 100 Years* (Agtlen, PA: Schiffer, 1998), 7.

58 Jacob Benignus Winslow, "Reflexions anatomiques sur les incommodités, infirmités, etc. qui arrivent au corps humain à l'occasion de certains attitudes & de certains habillements," in *Mémoires de mathématique et de physique: Histoire de l'Académie Royale des Sciences 1740*, published 1742, 59–65. Cited in Linder and Saltzman, 204. Linder and Saltzman do not make known the translator of this text. This is an excerpt of a speech by Winslow delivered before the

French Académie Royale des Sciences in 1740 in which he sharply criticized women's high-heeled shoes for their adverse impact on the wearers' health.

59 *Peter Camper, Dissertation sur la meilleure forme des souliers 1781*, 7, 46. Cited in Linder and Saltzman, 205. Translator unknown.

60 "The Fashions: Description of Fashion Plate," *Ladies' Treasury*, June 1, 1868, 85. Cited in Linder and Saltzman, 207. This was a British women's magazine.

61 Fordyce Barker, "Discussion," *Transactions of the American Gynecological Society* (1882) 7:261–263, 262. Cited in Linder and Saltzman, 201.

62 J. Goldthwait, et al., *Essentials of Body Mechanics in Health and Disease, 5th ed.* (Philadelphia: Lippincott, 1952), 295–96. Originally published 1934. This was a medical textbook. Cited in Linder and Saltzman, 213.

63 George Bankoff, *The Essential Eve: A Guide to Women's Perfection* (London: Cassell, 1952), 93–94. Cited in Cox, 82.

64 Carol Frey, "Foot Health and Shoewear for Women," *Clinical Orthopaedics and Related Research* (2000) 372:32–44.

65 Cox, 18.

66 Cox, 52.

67 Jonathan Walford, *The Seductive Shoe: Four Centuries of Fashion Footwear* (New York: Stewart, Tabori & Chang, 2007), 195.

68 Florence E. Ledger, *Put Your Foot Down: A Treatise on the History of Shoes* (Melksham: Colin Venton, 1976), 171. Cited in Cox, 86.

69 John T. Molloy, *The Woman's Dress for Success Book* (New York: Warner, 1977), 79, 35.

70 Sarah Baxter, "Fashion Victims Have Their Toes Trimmed to Fit Shoes," *Sunday Times* (London), August 10, 2003, available online at *www.timesonline.co.uk*.

71 As described on *www.ninewest.com*, August 9, 2009.

72 Simon Doonan, "Simon Says," *New York Observer*, July 27, 2009, 9.

73 *Exodus* 3:5.

74 *Deuteronomy* 25:5–10.

75 Catherine Hezser, "The Halitzah Shoe: Between Female Subjugation and Symbolic Emasculation," in *Nahshon*, 49.

76 In *Genesis Rabbah* 41:2, Rabbi Berekhyah says that Pharoah dared to approach the "shoe" of Sarai; In *Babylonian Kiddushin* 49a, a woman may reject a suitor on the grounds that she does not want "a shoe too large for my foot."

77 Ernest Jones, "Psycho-Analysis and Folklore," in *Essays in Applied Psycho-Analysis*, vol. 2 (New York: International Universities Press, 1964), 11. This paper was delivered in 1928.

78 Cited in James E. Crombie, "Shoe-Throwing at Weddings," *Folklore: A Quarterly Review of Myth, Tradition, Institution, & Custom, Being the Transactions of the Folk-Lore Society* (1895), vol. 6, 267.

79 Sigmund Freud, "Fetishism," in *The Standard Edition of the Complete Psychological Works of Sigmund Freud*, trans. James Strachey, vol. 11 (London: Hogarth, 1961), 154. "Fetishism" was written in 1927.

80 John C. Flügel, *The Psychology of Clothes* (London: Hogarth Press and the Institute of Psycho-Analysis, 1950), 27. Third printing. First published in 1930.

81 Havelock Ellis, *Studies in the Psychology of Sex*, vols. 1 and 2 (New York: Random House, 1936). Cited in Rossi, 142, 168.

82 Ernest Becker, *The Denial of Death* (New York: The Free Press, 1973), 237.

83 Sheila Jeffreys, *Beauty and Misogyny: Harmful Cultural Practices in the West* (London and New York: Routledge, 2005), 128.

84 Rossi, 94.

85   Rossi, 95.

86   Rossi, 91, 86, 90.

87   Rossi, 9.

88   Francis P. Magoun Jr. and Alexander H. Krappe, trans., "Aschenputtel," from *The Grimms' German Folk Tales* (Carbondale: Southern Illinois University Press, 1960), 86–92. In Alan Dundes, ed., *Cinderella: A Caseboook* (Wisconsin: University of Wisconsin Press, 1982, 1988), 27–29.

89   Paul Delarue, "From Perrault to Walt Disney: The Slipper of Cinderella," in Dundes, 110–111.

90   Freud, "Fetishism," 157.

91   The Western viewpoint, formed on the basis of missionary accounts and erotic literature, is nicely summarized by Valerie Steele in *Fetish: Fashion, Sex, and Power* (New York and Oxford: Oxford University Press, 1996), 92–95.

92   Dorothy Ko, *Every Step a Lotus: Shoes for Bound Feet* (Berkeley, Los Angeles, and London: University of California Press with the Bata Shoe Museum, 2001), 12.

93   Ko, 54, 63.

94   Ko, 104.

95   Susie Lan Cassel, "'. . . The Binding Altered Not Only My Feet But My Whole Character': Footbinding and First-World Feminism in Chinese American Literature." *Journal of Asian American Studies* (February 2007) 10.1:50–51.

96   Louisa Lim, "Painful Memories for China's Footbinding Survivors," National Public Radio, *Morning Edition*, March 29, 2007, transcript available on *http://www.npr.org*.

97 These stores include: in Berkeley, CA, The Walk Shop (*walkshop.com*); in Boston, MA, The Tannery (*thetannery.com*); in Chicago, IL, Hanig's Footwear (*hanigs.com*); in Great Neck, NY, The Clog Shop (*medshoes.com*); in New York, NY, Eneslow (*eneslow.com*), Harry's Shoes (*harrys-shoes.com*), and Tip Top Shoes (*tiptopshoes.com*); in Palo Alto and San Francisco, CA, Arthur Beren Shoes (*berenshoes.com*); in Pittsburgh, PA, Littles Shoes (*littlesshoes.com*); in Santa Fe, NM, Street Feet (*streetfeetsantafe.com*). If you are aware of additional shoe stores that provide excellent customer service and a wide range of stylish, sensible shoes, please email me at *leoratan@yahoo.com* so that I can add it in future editions of this book.

98 This is the conclusion of a study of 3,378 men and women from Framingham, MA, whose average age was 66. See Alyssa B. Dufour, et al., "Foot Pain: Is Current or Past Shoewear a Factor?" *Arthritis Care & Research* (October 2009) 61.10:1352–1358.

99 Coughlin, "Women's Shoe Wear and Foot Disorders."

100 Mark G. Mandato and Elizabeth Nester, "The Effects of Increasing Heel Height on Forefoot Peak Pressure," *Journal of the American Podiatric Medical Association* (February 1999) 89.2:75–80.

101 "Flip-Flops Be Gone! Give Your Feet a Break!" *ABC News*, August 22, 2007, available online at *www.hss.edu/newsroom_16785.asp*.

102 Call Eneslow, at 212-477-2300, for further information.

103 APMA, "New Study Compares Over-the-Counter Foot Inserts with Prescription Orthotics," June 23, 2009, available online at *www.apma.org*.

104 If you are aware of another shoe manufacturer not listed here that creates high-quality, sensible, stylish shoes, please email me at *leoratan@yahoo.com* so that I can add the information in future editions of this book.

Index

Achilles tendon, 17, 59, 108, 148

Alexander McQueen, 4

American Orthopaedic Foot & Ankle Society
    (AOFAS), 23, 25, 69, 74, 77, 78

American Podiatric Medical Association
    (APMA), 14, 16, 24, 74, 155

Andersen, Hans Christian, 28

André Courrèges, 116

arch of foot, 55–60

back pain, 60, 68, 104

ballet flats, 12, 149, 157

Bally, 42

Bankoff, George, 112

Barker, Fordyce, 111

Barneys New York, 118

Bata Shoe Museum (Toronto), 19, 95, 160

Baum, Frank L., 28

Becker, Ernest, *see* fetish object

Bernhard, Sandra, 51

Binet, Alfred, 121

Birkenstocks, 94, 116, 158

Blahnik, Manolo, *see* Manolo Blahnik

blisters, *see* foot, deformities, painful
    conditions

Bloomingdale's, 36

Botox, 77
    for face, 50, 89
    for feet, 89

Bradshaw, Carrie, 13, 27, 29–32, 39–40, 52

Brian Reyes, 3

Brogan, *see* historical shoes

Bruni-Sarkozy, Carla, 141

bunions, *see* foot, deformities, painful
        conditions

bunionettes, *see* foot, deformities, painful
        conditions

BunionSurvivor.com, 52, 80, 92

van Buren, Abigail, or "Dear Abby," 115

bursitis, 63

Bust magazine, 49

Butler, Judith, 123

California State University-San Marcos, 138

calluses, *see* foot, deformities, painful
        conditions

Campbell, Naomi, 4

Camper, Peter, 109

Chanel, 9, 20, 45, 76

Charles Jourdan, 38–39, 114

Chinese foot-binding, 133–139

Choo, Jimmy, *see* Jimmy Choo

chopine, *see* historical shoes

Christian Dior, 9, 113–114

Christian Louboutin, 9, 12, 19, 159

Cinderella, 11, 40–41, 130–133

"comfort" shoes, *see* shoes that are not "bad"

Copeland, Glenn, 23, 60

Coppola, Sofia, 141

corns, *see* foot, deformities, painful
    conditions

cosmetic surgery for feet
    complications from, 77–80
    foot narrowing, 77, 80
    toe shortening, 77, 80
    see also surgery for feet

Couric, Katie, 76

Courrèges, André, *see* André Courrèges

Cox, Caroline, 114

crackow, *see* historical shoes

cushioning inserted under ball of foot, 65–
    66, 75, 89–90, 144–145, 148, 152
    complications from, 90–91

Davis, Geena, 17

Delman, Herman, 114

The Denial of Death, 125

Dolce & Gabbana, 9

Doonan, Simon, 118

Dr. Scholl's, 154

Dreeben, Sharon, 78–79, 90–91

Dsquared2, 3

Double Indemnity, 113

Elle, 40

Ellis, Havelock, 124

Emilio Pucci, 3

Eneslow (New York City), 151, 161

feminism, feminist
    1968 protest of Miss America pageant, 48,
      50
    liberal strand of, 48–49
    not opposed to beauty, 21–22
    protest of oppressive beauty standards, 48
    psychoanalytic theory, *see Fetish object*
    radical strand of, 47
    suffragists, 104–105
    writing of Mary Wollstonecraft, *see*
      Wollstonecraft, Mary

femininity, pressure to adhere to rigid
    standard of, 16, 25, 47–51, 115

Ferragamo, Salvatore, 106, 114

fetish object
    Ernest Becker's theory of, 125–126
    feet as, 121–122
    feminist psychoanalytic theories of, 123
    John C. Flügel's theory of, 122–123
    Sigmund Freud's theory of, 121–122, 126
    Karl Marx's theory of, 121
    shoes as, 120–124, 126–127, 129

flappers, 105

flip-flops, 2, 20, 149
    as potentially dangerous, 12, 21
    as signifier of leisure, 95
    as signifier of sexuality, 95

Flügel, John C., *see* fetish object

Foot
    deformities, painful conditions
        blisters, 24, 40, 53, 69
        bunions, or "hallux valgus," 13–14,
            16–17, 22–24, 40, 42, 61–62, 68–
            70, 72, 75, 79–82, 84–87, 89,
            91–92, 147, 152, 154–155
        bunionettes, 14, 17, 23, 62, 70, 91,
            147
        calluses, 14, 24, 63–65, 68, 147
        corns, 14, 23–24, 63–65, 68, 110, 147
        hammertoes, 13, 17, 23, 63–64, 68–
            70, 72–73, 78–84, 87, 92, 147
        ingrown toenails, 14, 24, 69
        neuroma (Morton's Neuroma), 17,
            23, 66–69, 78, 147
        pinched nerve, 14, 66
        plantar fasciitis (heel pain), 21, 65–
            66, 68–69, 73, 149
    exercises, 72–73, 87
    pronation of, 22, 58, 60–62, 71, 144,
        154–155
    structure of, 55–60
    supination of, 60
Ford, Tom, see Tom Ford
Freud, Sigmund,
    on castration anxiety and fetish objects, see
        fetish object
    on Chinese footbinding, 134, 136
Frey, Carol, 14, 58, 69–73, 113, 147, 155

"girl culture," 49
gladiator sandals, 12
Glamour, 151
God, 29, 97, 119, 121
Go Fug Yourself (website), 4
Gold Cross shoes, 106–107
The Good Foot Book, 23
Grimm, Jacob and Wilhelm, 130
Gucci, 3

hallux valgus, *see* foot, deformities, painful
    conditions
hammertoes, *see* foot, deformities, painful
    conditions
Harper's Bazaar, 4, 19
Hebrew Bible, 119
heel pain, *see* foot, deformities, painful
    conditions
*Heights of Fashion: A History of the Elevated
    Shoe*, 19–20, 96, 160
Hepburn, Audrey, 141
Hepburn, Katharine, 141
Hervé Léger by Max Azria, 3
high-heeled shoes
    as affirmation of gender identity, 50, 124–
        125, 127
    as cause of accidents, 23
    as cause of change in posture, 5, 51, 129
    as cause of foot deformity, 17
    as cause of excruciating pain, 15, 24, 110
    ease of shopping for, 12, 32–33

inability to walk in, 3, 11–12, 18, 44–46, 52–53, 109, 112

insane prices of, 10, 19, 31, 159–161

looking foolish in, 52

lying about how uncomfortable they are, 43–45

as phallic symbol, 123–124, 128, 137

as signifier of strength, 49, 51, 138

similarities with Chinese foot-binding, 137–139

stilettos, 4, 10–11, 13, 17, 19, 21, 24, 27, 40, 91, 96, 114–117, 141, 148, 151

tacones, 50

as vulval symbol, 122–123, 137

hip pain, 68

historical shoes

brogan, 102–103

chopine, 97–99

of Louis XIV, 99–100

qabqab, 96

patten, 101–102

platform, 106

poulaine, or *crackow*, 96–97, 115

shoe rose, 100

slap sole, 101

stilettos, *see High-heeled shoes*

wedge, 106

winklepicker, 115

Hoed, Elyse, 84

Hospital for Special Surgery (New York City), 16

ingrown toenails, *see* foot, deformities, painful conditions

Institute Beauté, 77, 89

International Aesthetic Foot Society (IAFS), 89–90

J. Crew, 33

Jimmy Choo, 9, 18, 41–42, 159

Jong, Erica, 93

Jourdan, Charles, *see* Charles Jourdan

Juvéderm, 89

Kennedy Onassis, Jacqueline, 141

Kerber, Betty, 87

Kershaw, Julian, 141

Knee pain, 60, 68, 104

Ko, Dorothy, 135–136, 138

von Krafft-Ebing, Richard Freiherr, 121

Lacan, Jacques, 123

Ladies' Home Journal, 105

Lan Cassel, Susie, 138

Lancet, 104

Lautin, Everett, 77, 89–90

de Lauretis, Teresa, 123

Leder, Bobbi, 85

Levine, Suzanne, 76–78, 80, 89–90

Lim, Louisa, 139

Louboutin, Christian, *see* Christian
    Louboutin
Louis XIV's shoes, *see* historical shoes
love of shoes, 32–39

Manolo Blahnik, 3, 20, 29–30, 39, 41, 45,
    76, 79, 118, 151, 159
Marcdante, Mary, 52–53, 80–81, 92
Marcos, Imelda, 27
Marx, Karl, *see* fetish object
Marzouka-Losito, Cynthia, 90
McCartney, Stella, *see* Stella McCartney
McDowell, Colin, 97
Miller, Sienna, 141
Miu Miu, 3
Molloy, John T., 116–117
Monroe, Marilyn, 115
Morgan, Jessica, 4
Morton's Neuroma, *see* foot, deformities,
    painful conditions
Moses, 119

National Public Radio, 139
National Shoe Manufacturers' Association, 115
neuroma, *see* foot, deformities, painful
    conditions
new shoes, 53–54
New York Giants, 16
New York Mets, 16
New Yorker, 51

New York Times, 70, 76, 104
New York Observer, 76
Nine West, 118

Obama, Michelle, 141
O'Neal, Tatum, 29, 31
orthopedic shoes, 13, 31, 76, 79
orthopedist, definition of, 74
orthotics, 22, 25, 60, 62, 65–66, 68, 90–92,
    144, 146, 149, 153–157
Oscar de la Renta, 9

Parker, Sarah Jessica, 29, 40
patten, *see* historical shoes
pedorthist, definition of, 74
Perrault, Charles, 133
pinched nerve, *see* foot, deformities, painful
    conditions
pinup models, 107, 115
plantar fasciitis, *see* foot, deformities, painful
    conditions
Playboy, 115
podiatrist, definition of, 73–74
pointed-toe shoes, as cause of foot deformity,
    6, 14–16
Positano, Rock, 16, 23–24, 77–80, 90, 149
The Postman Always Rings Twice, 113
Posture Dynamics, 154
Poulaine, *see* Historical shoes
Powerstep, 154

Prada, 3, 14, 45–46, 158
pronation, *see* foot
prostitutes, 95, 98, 103
Pucci, Emilio, *see* Emilio Pucci

Qabqab, *see* historical shoes

"The Red Shoes" (Hans Christian Andersen), 28–29
de la Renta, Oscar, *see* Oscar de la Renta
Reed, Donna, 49
Reyes, Brian, *see* Brian Reyes
Rodarte, 3
Roosevelt, Eleanor, 21, 128
Rossi, William A., 127–129
Rothweiler, Brittney, 142
RuPaul, 49

von Sacher-Masoch, Leopold, 121
de Sade, Marquis, 121
Saint Laurent, Yves, *see* Yves Saint Laurent
Saks Fifth Avenue, 9, 11, 13
Salvation Army, 13, 127
Sand, George, 102
Sarandon, Susan, 17
Sawyer, Diane, 76
Schwartz, Robert, 161
Schwartz, Suze Yalof, 151
Scoop (New York City), 41

Sculptra, 89–90
Semmelhack, Elizabeth, 19–20, 94–96, 99–101, 160
"sensible" shoes, *see* shoes that are not "bad"
September 11, 2001, 19–20
Sex and the City (movie and tv show), 13, 29–32, 52
The Sex Life of the Foot and Shoe, 127
sexual exhibitionism
    in fashion, 93–94
    in footwear, 94–96, 117–118
Shoes: Fashion and Fantasy, 97
shoe roses, *see* historical shoes
shoes, structure of
combination-lasted, 71
    too narrow, 71
    too small, 69–70
    wide-sized, 71, 142
shoes that are not "bad"
    "comfort" shoes, 25, 55, 125
    customization of, 151–152
    empowerment in, 161–162
    looking good in, 141, 161–162
    "sensible" shoes, 6, 21, 27, 50, 91, 106–107, 124–128, 141
    shopping for, 142–151, 158
slap sole, *see* historical shoes
Solemate, 152
Solomon, Stan, 23
Spenco, 154
Stanwyck, Barbara, 113
Stella McCartney, 160–161

Sternbergh, Adam, 58
stilettos, see high-heeled shoes
Stuart Weitzman, 158–159
SuperFeet, 154
supination, see foot
surgery for feet
    advice about, 92
    cosmetic, see cosmetic surgery for feet
    for bunion, 16, 79–81
    for hammertoe, 17, 79–80
    inability to move toes as a result of, 86–87
    surgery gone bad, 77–78, 81–88
    toes removed as a result of, 87–88

Talley, André Leon, 5
The Tannery (Boston), 142
Tip Top Shoes (New York City), 144
Today Show, 76
Tom Ford, 20
Toronto Blue Jays, 23
Turner, Lana, 113
Twiggy, 116

University of California, Los Angeles, 14

Valentino, 9
Venus in Furs, 121
Vivienne Westwood, 4

Vivier, Roger, 114
Vogue, 5, 76, 114, 141

The Walk Shop (Berkeley, CA), 141
Walford, Jonathan, 115
Walters, Barbara, 76
Washington Post, 105
Wasserman, Danny, 144
Weitzman, Stuart, see Stuart Weitzman
Westwood, Vivienne, see Vivienne Westwood
Winfrey, Oprah, 76
Winslet, Kate, 141
Winslow, Jacob, 109
Wintour, Anna, 76, 141
Witherspoon, Reese, 141
The Wizard of Oz, 28
Wollstonecraft, Mary, 101
The Women's Dress for Success Book, 116
Women's Wear Daily, 118

Youner, Johanna, 16, 23, 79, 91, 149–150,
        154–155, 159
Yves Saint Laurent, 9, 11

Acknowledgments

I AM FORTUNATE to be surrounded by intelligent, interesting, and—yes—stylish women who are level-headed about high-heeled shoes. Thank you to my superb agent, Jennifer Lyons, and to the wonder women I worked with at Seven Stories: editor Crystal Yakacki, publicity director Ruth Weiner, and managing editor Veronica Liu. Thank you to Vanessa Davis for capturing the fun, fantasy, and folly of women's footwear. I also owe a huge thank you to the mighty men who designed and stitched this book: Jon Gilbert, operations director, and Stewart Cauley, designer. And to Dan Simon, publisher and visionary of Seven Stories: Thank you for empathizing with women and putting yourself in our shoes—although I would never wish on you the pain of a pointy-toed stiletto.

About the Author

LEORA TANENBAUM writes about the lives of women and girls (*www.leoratanenbaum.com*). She is the author of *Slut! Growing Up Female with a Bad Reputation, Catfight: Rivalries Among Women—From Diets to Dating, From the Boardroom to the Delivery Room,* and *Taking Back God: American Women Rising Up for Religious Equality.* She is a blogger for the *Huffington Post* and lives in New York City.

If you want to contact Leora with questions, comments, or rants about cage boots and other senseless shoe trends, please email her at *leoratan@yahoo.com*.

About Seven Stories Press

SEVEN STORIES PRESS is an independent book publisher based in New York City, with distribution throughout the United States, Canada, England, and Australia. We publish works of the imagination by such writers as Nelson Algren, Russell Banks, Octavia E. Butler, Ani DiFranco, Assia Djebar, Ariel Dorfman, Coco Fusco, Barry Gifford, Hwang Sok-yong, Lee Stringer, and Kurt Vonnegut, to name a few, together with political titles by voices of conscience, including the Boston Women's Health Collective, Noam Chomsky, Angela Y. Davis, Human Rights Watch, Derrick Jensen, Ralph Nader, Loretta Napoleoni, Gary Null, Project Censored, Barbara Seaman, Alice Walker, Gary Webb, and Howard Zinn, among many others. Seven Stories Press believes publishers have a special responsibility to defend free speech and human rights, and to celebrate the gifts of the human imagination, wherever we can. For additional information, visit www.sevenstories.com.